**5th Edition**

# Complete Math Review for the Pharmacy Technician

William A. Hopkins Jr.

**William A. Hopkins Jr., PharmD, RPh, FACA**
President
Clinical Pharmacy Consultants of North Georgia
Big Canoe, Georgia

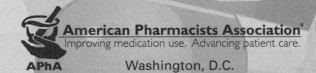

**American Pharmacists Association®**
Improving medication use. Advancing patient care.

APhA

Washington, D.C.

Managing Editor: John Fedor
Design and Composition: Circle Graphics
Cover Design: Scott Neitzke, APhA Integrated Design and Production Center
Proofreading: Publications Professionals

Published by the American Pharmacists Association
2215 Constitution Avenue, N.W.
Washington, DC 20037-2985
www.pharmacist.com   www.pharmacylibrary.com

To comment on this book via e-mail, send your message to the publisher at aphabooks@aphanet.org.

**Library of Congress Cataloging-in-Publication Data**

Names: Hopkins, William A., Jr. (William Alexander), 1947- author. | American
  Pharmacists Association, publisher.
Title: Complete math review for the pharmacy technician / William A. Hopkins
  Jr.
Other titles: APhA pharmacy technician training series.
Description: 5th edition. | Washington, DC : American Pharmacists
  Association, [2019] | Series: APhA pharmacy technician training series
Identifiers: LCCN 2019006907 | ISBN 9781582123141
Subjects: | MESH: Drug Dosage Calculations | Mathematics | Pharmaceutical
  Preparations–administration & dosage
Classification: LCC RS57 | NLM QV 748 | DDC 615/.1401513–dc23 LC record available at https://lccn.loc.gov/2019006907

## How To Order This Book

Online: www.pharmacist.com/shop
By phone: 800-878-0729 (770-280-0085 from outside the United States)
VISA®, MasterCard®, and American Express® cards accepted.

*To my loving parents, William and Mary Frances,*
*to my wonderful children, Bill, Kim, Angie, Nadia, and Abby*
*and my grandchildren, Carly, Stella, Kai, Hadley, Beckett,*
*and Keylana, and to my precious wife, Patricia,*
*for her love and dedication.*

# Contents

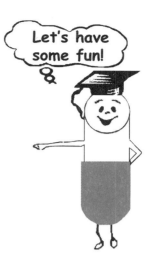

# Preface

Have you ever said **"I can't stand math"**? For five decades, I have heard numerous pharmacists, technicians, nurses, and other healthcare practitioners make this statement.

I have personally made similar comments. Unfortunately, most of my teachers were unable to make math interesting, practical, or fun. The aforementioned are reasons I finally decided to write a textbook that is easy to understand, practical, and entertaining.

By now, you have probably noticed I am writing to you personally and not in the "third person." It is important to me that you relax and know that I recognize the barriers and fears you are experiencing in learning pharmacy calculations.

I will become your personal tutor and cheerleader throughout this book and hopefully will prove to you that math can be easy and enjoyable. More importantly, I want you to learn for life and not just for certification or for final exams.

This textbook has been written in a self-instructional format, so you can use it either while studying alone or in support of a formal course. It will also serve as a reference book throughout your pharmacy career.

When teaching math, I believe in the old acronym *K.I.S.S.,* which stands for "keep it simple, sweetie." In sticking with this approach, I promise to keep math at an uncomplicated level. In fact, you won't need to remember your algebra, geometry, trigonometry, or calculus to be successful with my techniques. Most problems in this book will be worked in the same manner, using a simple ratio and proportion process.

In addition, I avoid formulas when teaching for several reasons. First, people tend to forget formulas or to become confused when using them, leading to potential disasters. Second, many mistakes are made by people who are just plugging numbers into equations without understanding the logic behind the formulas. I want you to be totally confident that your answer is correct when solving each and every problem.

We will start this book by performing the most basic math functions and slowly progress to more challenging issues. It has been my experience that students who have difficulty with math frequently do not have a grasp of the fundamental concepts and then progress too quickly to the tougher questions.

With this in mind, **please** *master the basics and do not skip or hurry through early sections*. **Always** contact your instructor if you are having a problem with any concept, no matter how basic it may be. Each chapter will contain questions and examples that have nothing to do with pharmacy practice. The purpose of this is to help you relate what you are learning in this book to everyday life.

By so doing, you will improve all of your math skills, not just those related to being a pharmacy technician. Finally, there will be a cumulative examination that will enable you to assess how far you have progressed.

In this fifth edition, I have added 100 new questions drawn directly from manufacturers' drug package inserts.

**Good luck** in your career in pharmacy and in all other future endeavors. Now let's get started with a positive attitude about math and have a little fun.

# Acknowledgments

I wish to thank the American Pharmacists Association for its leadership of our profession and for giving me the opportunity to write this textbook.

A special thanks to Dr. Loyd Allen, editor in chief of the *International Journal of Pharmaceutical Compounding,* who has graciously permitted the use of innovative formulas from his publication. I am also grateful to many pharmaceutical companies for the use of their package inserts and labels.

# Back to Basics

Welcome to the second step in learning about pharmaceutical calculations. The first step was reading the Preface, which you probably skipped if you are like most of my students! I will wait a few minutes while you go back and read those very important pages.

Now that you have mastered Step One, let's start learning the important fundamentals of math necessary for future chapters and for your work in pharmacy.

## Arabic and Roman Numerals

All of you are familiar with the "Arabic" system of notation, the basic ten figures 0, 1, 2, 3, 4, 5, 6, 7, 8, 9. These figures are arranged in various orders with different values assigned to the digits according to the location they occupy in a row. An example would be the numbers 21 and 210. You all know from your first-grade education that the "2" in 21 has a value of 20, but in 210 the "2" stands for 200.

*Here come the Romans!!!*

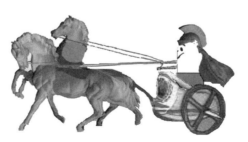

There is another system of notation known as "Roman numerals" that is a lot older than I am! This system dates back thousands of years and is still being used by some practitioners today. You are probably asking yourself why this is occurring. The primary reason is because of an ancient system of measurement known as the "apothecaries' system."

This method requires the use of Roman numerals. An example would be writing the abbreviation of 6 grains, which is "gr.vi." The apothecaries' system is discouraged in contemporary pharmacy practice, but you need to understand Roman numerals because they still appear on many prescriptions and compounding formulas.

The Roman system utilizes eight letters to designate numbers. (Throughout this book, my assistant, Wily Willie, will point out important things for you.) Before you continue, take a little time and memorize these Roman numerals and their Arabic equivalents:

| $\frac{1}{2}$ | = | SS | | |
|---|---|---|---|---|
| 1 | = | I | or | i |
| 5 | = | V | or | v |
| 10 | = | X | or | x |
| 50 | = | L | or | l |
| 100 | = | C | or | c |
| 500 | = | D | or | d |
| 1000 | = | M | or | m |

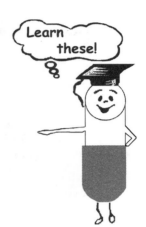

Learn these!

Now that you have mastered Roman numerals, it is time to create Arabic numbers from Roman numerals and vice versa. Unfortunately, I have bad news for you, because the two systems are very different in how they work.

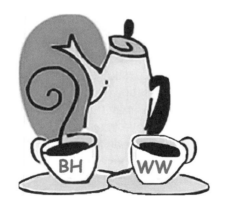

For example, the number 40 cannot be written as XXXX, nor can the number 15 be written as VVV.

### Why?

Because there are eight rules of Roman numerals you have to learn before we continue.

**So get to work and memorize the rules on the next page while Wily Willie and I take a break.**

# Roman Numeral Rules

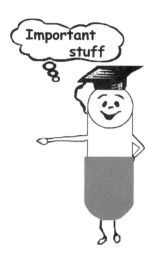

1. When a letter is repeated, its value is repeated.

   II = 1 + 1 = 2 and XXX = 10 + 10 + 10 = 30

   *So, you ask,"Why isn't XXXX equal to 40?"*

   *Keep reading, and you will figure it out.*

2. A letter cannot be repeated more than three times.

   *So XXXX is not equal to 40, and VVVVV is not equal to 25. But what about VVV?*

3. V, L, and D are never repeated.

   *This explains why VVV is not equal to 15, nor is VV equal to 10.*

4. When a **smaller** numeral (letter) is placed **before** a **larger** numeral, it is **subtracted** from the larger numeral.

   IV = 4      IX = 9      XL = 40      CD = 400      CM = 900

5. When a **smaller** numeral is placed **after** a **larger** numeral, it is **added** to the larger numeral.

   VI = 6      XI = 11      LX = 60      MC = 1100      MD = 1500

6. V, L, and D are never subtracted from larger numbers.

   *So VL is not equal to 45, and LM is not equal to 950.*

7. Never subtract more than one numeral.

   *So IIX is not equal to 8, and XXXC is not equal to 70.*

8. Use I before V and X only (the next two highest numerals). The same is true for X and C (i.e., X before L and C; C before D and M).

   IV = 4 and IX = 9 **but** IC is **not** equal to 99

   XC = 90 **but** XM is **not** equal to 990

# PRACTICE

*Please* work all problems in this book with a **pencil** so corrections can be easily made.

**1.** Write the corresponding Arabic or Roman numbers for the following:

(a) CC    =          (e) XL    =          (i)  XII   =

(b) LL    =          (f)  VD    =          (j)  IIC   =

(c) MMM =          (g) LV    =

(d) CCCC =          (h) IM    =

If you had trouble with a–j, restudy rules 1–8 before continuing.

(k) XXII   =          (q) DXV   =          (w) 47   =

(l)  LI     =          (r)  XXIX  =          (x) 62   =

(m) CX    =          (s) CDXLV =          (y) 480  =

(n) CL    =          (t)  XIVI   =          (z) 1999 =

(o) LXVI  =          (u) 18     =

(p) MIV   =          (v) 34     =

The answers to all problems can be found in the **Answer Key** beginning on page 253.

## Fractions

A fraction indicates a portion of a whole number. There are two types of fractions discussed in this chapter. They are the **common** fractions and the **decimal** fractions. Let's first look at common fractions.

## Common Fractions

A common fraction is an expression of division with one number placed over another. Examples of common fractions are $\frac{1}{2}$ and $\frac{3}{4}$.

The bottom number is referred to as the **denominator**, and the top number is the **numerator**. In these examples, the numerators are the numbers 1 and 3, and the denominators are the numbers 2 and 4. The denominator represents the number of parts that the whole number is divided into. In the example $\frac{1}{2}$, the whole number is divided into 2 parts. In the example $\frac{3}{4}$, the whole number is divided into 4 parts. The numerator tells us how many of those parts we are concerned with.

*Are you confused?*

Let's take the first example, $\frac{1}{2}$, and discuss it. All of you know what $\frac{1}{2}$ means. If I said you have $\frac{1}{2}$ dollar, you know you have 50 cents. You knew that from everyday experiences. But even though you knew the answer, did you really understand the concept? It is important to have a thorough understanding of how fractions work before we get to Chapter 3 and start learning ratios and proportions. So take a few minutes and think about the definition of a common fraction and how it relates to the dollar example.

If the denominator of $\frac{1}{2}$ is 2, this means that the total number is divided into 2 parts. In the case of a dollar, the 100 cents are divided into 2 parts, each containing 50 cents. The numerator tells us how many of those parts we are concerned with. So with a numerator of 1, we will have 1 of the 2 parts, each containing 50 cents.

How many cents would be in $\frac{3}{4}$ of a dollar? Think about this based on our discussion, not on what is in your "memory bank." The denominator is 4, meaning the 100 cents in a dollar are broken into 4 parts, each containing 25 cents. The numerator is 3, which means you are concerned with 3 parts, or a total of 75 cents (i.e., $3 \times 25 = 75$).

*Now that you think this is so easy, why don't you try one?*

**Question:**  How many cents would be in $\frac{13}{20}$ of a dollar?

*(OK, OK, I had the easy ones, but see if you can solve this in the space below before looking at the solution.)*

**Solution:**   1 dollar is equal to 100 cents. 100 cents divided by 20 (the denominator) equals 5 cents per part. Multiply 5 cents per part by 13 (i.e., the numerator) and the answer is 65 cents.

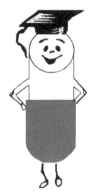

## Types of Common Fractions

In the previous section, we were discussing common fractions in a form sometimes referred to as **proper** fractions. These are fractions where the numerator is smaller than the denominator, that is, $\frac{1}{2}, \frac{3}{4}$, etc. There are several other types of fractions you need to know.

**Improper fractions** are fractions where the numerator is larger than the denominator. They are often used when adding, subtracting, multiplying, and dividing with fractions.

***Examples:***   $\frac{9}{7}$      $\frac{13}{12}$      $\frac{37}{18}$

**Mixed fractions** are combinations of whole numbers and proper fractions.

***Examples:***    $1\frac{1}{2}$ and $3\frac{3}{4}$

> *Mixed fractions must be converted to improper fractions before calculating.*

## Calculating with Fractions

Before calculating with fractions, make sure all mixed fractions are changed to improper fractions. This is easily done by simply multiplying the whole number by the denominator and then adding the numerator and placing the resulting number over the denominator.

***Example:***    To change $4\frac{1}{2}$ to an improper fraction, multiply the whole number (4) by the denominator (2), which equals 8. Now add the numerator (1) to give the number 9. Simply place the 9 over the original denominator (2) and your answer is $\frac{9}{2}$. So, $4\frac{1}{2}$ is equal to $\frac{9}{2}$.

*Now you need to try one.*

***Question:***    Convert this mixed fraction to an improper fraction: $12\frac{5}{8} =$ **?**

***Solution:***    Multiply 12 times the denominator (8) = 96
Add 96 to the numerator (5) = 101
Place the 101 over the original denominator (8)
And the answer is $12\frac{5}{8} = \frac{101}{8}$

## Multiplying Fractions

I am starting with **multiplication** because it is the easiest process of all. To multiply fractions, be sure to convert all whole numbers to improper fractions.

***Example:***    5    =    $\frac{5}{1}$

Make sure all mixed fractions are converted to improper fractions as well.

***Example:***    $2\frac{1}{2}$    =    $\frac{5}{2}$

Now all you have to do is multiply the numerators by each other and do the same for the denominators. Let's use these examples to multiply 5 by $2\frac{1}{2}$.

***Solution:*** $\quad 5 \quad \times \quad 2\frac{1}{2} \quad = \quad$ **?** $\quad$ *(Convert these to improper fractions.)*

$\qquad\qquad\quad \frac{5}{1} \quad \times \quad \frac{5}{2} \quad = \quad \frac{25}{2}$ *(Multiply numerators and denominators.)*

> The answer $\frac{25}{2}$ is correct, but the proper way of reporting this answer is in the form of a mixed fraction, or $12\frac{1}{2}$. To calculate the mixed fraction, simply divide the numerator (25) by the denominator (2), which gives you 12 with a remainder of 1. Make sure you put the remainder (1) over the denominator (2).

**NOTE**

***Tag, it's your turn to try one!*** $\qquad$ Multiply $5\frac{7}{8}$ times $\frac{3}{5}$.

***Solution:*** $\quad 5\frac{7}{8} \quad \times \quad \frac{3}{5} \quad = \quad$ **?**

$\qquad\qquad\quad \frac{47}{8} \quad \times \quad \frac{3}{5} \quad = \quad$ **?**

$\qquad\qquad\quad \frac{47}{8} \quad \times \quad \frac{3}{5} \quad = \quad \frac{141}{40} \quad = \quad 3\frac{21}{40}$

***Now why don't we try to put these fractions into a real-world problem?***

***Example:*** $\quad$ Yesterday I bought a box of 6 microwave popcorn packets. I noticed that each packet weighed $6\frac{3}{4}$ ounces. How much did the entire box weigh?

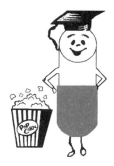

***Solution:*** $\quad 6\frac{3}{4} \quad \times \quad 6 \quad = \quad$ **?**

$\qquad\qquad\quad \frac{27}{4} \quad \times \quad \frac{6}{1} \quad = \quad \frac{162}{4} \quad = \quad 40\frac{2}{4}$ ounces

> Whenever possible, try to reduce fractions to the lowest terms. In this example, the answer $40\frac{2}{4}$ is correct, but the more cosmetically correct answer is $40\frac{1}{2}$. To reduce the fraction $\frac{2}{4}$ to lowest terms, divide the numerator and denominator by the highest number that will divide evenly into each number. In this case, the best number is 2.
>
> $$\frac{2 \div 2}{4 \div 2} = \frac{1}{2}$$ $\quad$ Your final answer will become $40\frac{1}{2}$ ounces.

**NOTE**

## Dividing Fractions

Dividing fractions is almost as easy as multiplying, but there is one big difference. When you divide fractions, you will do everything just like you were multiplying until you get to the last step. Before you multiply the numerators and denominators, you need to invert the divisor (the number you're going to divide by). Let's look at an example.

$$\frac{7}{12} \div 5 = \textbf{?}$$

$$\frac{7}{12} \div \frac{5}{1} = \textbf{?}$$

As you can see, the process so far is the same. Now for the big difference. In division, you invert the divisor before multiplying. I like to change the sign from (÷) to (×) when I invert the divisor. This is how it looks: $\frac{7}{12} \times \frac{1}{5} = \frac{7}{60}$

One of the most important math skills is **estimating**. Frequently, errors can be avoided if practitioners simply estimate correct answers. In this example, we were dividing a number with a value less than 1 by 5. It is easy to predict that the answer will be a small number (i.e., less than 1). If you were to make a math error and not invert the divisor in this problem, your answer would be almost 3.

*It's time again for you to show me how smart you are!*

**Question:**   Now I just bought a 20-ounce box of Cheerios®. How many meals can I eat out of this box if I eat $3\frac{1}{3}$ ounces of Cheerios every morning for breakfast? (Write your answer below before looking at the solution.)

**Solution:**   Did you **estimate** your answer before working this problem? If not, you are hopeless.               Just kidding!

Learning to estimate is hard to do, but take my word, it is well worth the effort. I estimated by saying that I have 20 ounces divided by about 3, so the correct answer is approximately 6 or 7 (plus or minus a few Cheerios).

$$20 \div 3\frac{1}{3} = \mathbf{?}$$
$$\frac{20}{1} \div \frac{10}{3} = \mathbf{?}$$
$$\frac{20}{1} \times \frac{3}{10} = \frac{60}{10} = \frac{6}{1} = 6 \text{ servings of Cheerios}$$

## Adding and Subtracting Fractions

Adding and subtracting fractions requires more work than multiplying and dividing. When adding and subtracting, you must find a common denominator for every fraction. This process must be done before you can proceed with calculating the answer. In solving for a **common denominator**, remember that the fraction will be exactly the same if you multiply or divide the numerator and denominator by the same number.

**Example:**   Multiply the numerator and denominator in the fraction $\frac{1}{2}$ by 5. Your answer is $\frac{5}{10}$. You all know that $\frac{5}{10}$ is the same as $\frac{1}{2}$, so the fractions are equal. If you took the fraction $\frac{7}{21}$ and divided the numerator and denominator by 7, you would have the fraction $\frac{1}{3}$. This means that $\frac{7}{21}$ and $\frac{1}{3}$ are equal fractions. Now let's solve for **common denominators** and start adding and subtracting fractions.

**Question:**   Add the following fractions: $\frac{5}{8} + \frac{1}{6} + \frac{2}{3} = \mathbf{?}$

*Think about the steps involved.*

**Step 1.** Make sure all numbers are proper or improper fractions (no mixed fractions).

**Step 2.** Find common denominators for all fractions. Simply take multiples of the "largest" of the 3 denominators until you come up with a number that all denominators will divide into an *even* number of times. In this example, the largest denominator is 8. Multiples of 8 are 16, 24, 32, 40, 48, 56, etc.

Which of these numbers is the lowest number that all 3 denominators will divide into an even number of times?

The answer is 24.

This means 24 is our lowest common denominator (LCD). The number 48 would also be OK, but higher numbers create more work and greater chances of making errors.

**Step 3.** Create new fractions that all have the same common denominator. Remember, earlier I told you that the "value" of fractions does not change if you multiply or divide both the numerator and denominator by the "same" number.

Now let's change all the fractions so they all have denominators of 24.
$\frac{5}{8} = \frac{?}{24}$ (The new denominator, 24, is 3 times larger than the 8 in $\frac{5}{8}$. If the new denominator is 3 times larger, then you need to also multiply the numerator by 3 to keep the fraction the same. So $\frac{5}{8}$ equals $\frac{15}{24}$.)

*Now you solve for $\frac{1}{6}$ and $\frac{2}{3}$.*

*Solution:* $\frac{1}{6} = \frac{?}{24}$      *Solution:* $\frac{2}{3} = \frac{?}{24}$
$\frac{1}{6} = \frac{4}{24}$                    $\frac{2}{3} = \frac{16}{24}$

**Step 4.** Add or subtract the numerators and place them over the common denominator.

**DO NOT add the denominators.**    $\frac{15}{24} + \frac{4}{24} + \frac{16}{24} = \frac{?}{24} = \frac{35}{24}$

**Step 5.** Reduce the answer to lowest terms or to a mixed fraction.
$\frac{35}{24} = 1\frac{11}{24}$

*It's show time! Try to solve this one.*

**Question:** My Uncle Dudley is a farmer. Last year he sold his corn crop to 3 different merchants. One merchant bought $\frac{3}{16}$ of Uncle Dudley's crop, another bought $\frac{1}{8}$, and the third merchant bought $\frac{13}{24}$ of the crop. How much of the total crop did they buy?

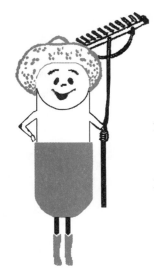

**Solution:** Step 1. All numbers are proper fractions.

Step 2. The common denominator is a multiple of 24 and is 48.

Step 3. Create new fractions with a denominator of 48:

$$\frac{3}{16} = \frac{9}{48}$$

$$\frac{13}{24} = \frac{26}{48}$$

$$\frac{1}{8} = \frac{6}{48}$$

Step 4. Add the numerators and place them over the common denominator:

$$\frac{9}{48} + \frac{26}{48} + \frac{6}{48} = \frac{?}{48} = \frac{41}{48}$$

Step 5. Already reduced to lowest terms.

**Question:** Now that you think you have mastered this process, why don't you tell me how much of Uncle Dudley's crop was left over after the merchants took their $\frac{41}{48}$.

**Solution:** Step 1. The total crop would be equal to all the parts (i.e., $\frac{48}{48}$, which is 1).

Step 2. The common denominator is 48.

Step 3. Both fractions, $\frac{48}{48}$ and $\frac{41}{48}$, have the same denominator.

Step 4. Subtract the numerators: $\frac{48}{48} - \frac{41}{48} = \frac{?}{48} = \frac{7}{48}$

Step 5. Already reduced to lowest terms. My uncle had $\frac{7}{48}$ of his crop left.

# PRACTICE

**2.** Multiply and reduce answers to lowest terms.

(a) $7 \times \frac{1}{12} = $ **?**   (d) $\frac{1}{500} \times 5 = $ **?**

(b) $\frac{3}{5} \times \frac{1}{5} = $ **?**   (e) $8\frac{3}{4} \times \frac{3}{120} = $ **?**

(c) $1\frac{1}{6} \times 2\frac{1}{2} = $ **?**

**3.** Divide and reduce answers to lowest terms.

(a) $\frac{3}{5} \div \frac{4}{5} = $ **?**   (d) $11 \div 3\frac{3}{4} = $ **?**

(b) $19\frac{1}{4} \div 3 = $ **?**   (e) $\frac{1}{8} \div 8 = $ **?**

(c) $\frac{1}{50} \div \frac{1}{200} = $ **?**

**4.** Add and reduce to lowest terms.

(a) $\frac{3}{8} + \frac{5}{16} = $ **?**

(b) $\frac{9}{13} + \frac{1}{3} = $ **?**

(c) $1\frac{5}{8} + 3\frac{3}{4} + 5\frac{3}{10} = $ **?**

(d) $10\frac{1}{2} + 5 + 6\frac{1}{3} = $ **?**

(e) $3\frac{2}{3} + 5\frac{1}{2} + \frac{5}{11} = $ **?**

**5.** Subtract and reduce to lowest terms.

(a) $\frac{4}{5} - \frac{3}{10} = $ **?**   (d) $\frac{3}{100} - \frac{1}{150} = $ **?**

(b) $5\frac{1}{12} - \frac{2}{3} = $ **?**   (e) $7\frac{2}{5} - \frac{2}{3} = $ **?**

(c) $11\frac{3}{4} - 9\frac{1}{2} = $ **?**

**6.** During the past few weeks I have purchased bananas on four different occasions. The weights were $\frac{3}{4}$ pound, $\frac{1}{2}$ pound, 2 pounds, and $1\frac{5}{8}$ pounds. How many pounds of bananas did I buy?

**7.** From your answer in Question 6, how many pounds of bananas have I consumed if I still have $1\frac{1}{2}$ pounds of uneaten bananas?

*OK, OK, so you're getting tired of bananas and Cheerios! Let's try a few of these problems and relate them to your career in pharmacy. Please note that the math is the same. We will only change the units to pharmaceutical and medical terms.*

**8.** A pharmacist buys sulfur powder at different times in quantities of $\frac{3}{8}$ pound, $1\frac{1}{2}$ pounds, $\frac{3}{16}$ pound, and 2 pounds. How much sulfur did she buy?

**9.** Using your answer from Question 8, how much sulfur would remain if the pharmacy technician compounded three prescriptions of mange powder, each containing $1\frac{1}{4}$ pounds of sulfur?

**10.** A bottle of children's cough syrup contains 24 teaspoons of medication. If the dose of the syrup for a 6-year-old is $\frac{3}{4}$ teaspoon, how many doses are in the bottle?

**11.** A cardiac patient taking $\frac{1}{150}$ grain nitroglycerin tablets took two tablets in the morning, one in the afternoon, and two in the evening. How many grains of nitroglycerin did the patient receive?

**12.** A prescription for 30 capsules requires a total of $\frac{3}{16}$ ounce of a potent narcotic. How much of the narcotic is contained in each capsule?

*The answers to all problems can be found in the **Answer Key** beginning on page 253.*

# Decimal Fractions

Decimals are fractions with a denominator of any multiple of 10 (e.g., 10, 100, 1000, 10,000). Decimal fractions differ from the common fractions we previously discussed in that decimal fractions signify the denominator with a decimal point placed to the left of the numerator. This probably doesn't make a whole lot of sense, so let me give you several examples.

**Example:**   $\frac{9}{10}$ written as a decimal fraction is 0.9.

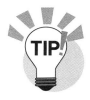

*The first place to the right of the decimal signifies tenths, the next place signifies hundredths, the next thousandths, then ten thousandths, etc. Always place a zero to the left of the decimal point if there is not a whole number occupying that position. Let's look at 0.35 and 0.00487. The example $\frac{9}{10}$ is written 0.9 and is read "nine-tenths." In the case of a mixed fraction like $3\frac{1}{100}$, you would write it as 3.01 and read it as "three and one-hundredth."*

**Example:**   $\frac{125}{1000}$ written as a decimal fraction is 0.125.

Would a zero to the right of 0.125 change the value of this decimal? The answer is *NO* because 0.1250 would be $\frac{1250}{10000}$, so when it is reduced it becomes $\frac{125}{1000}$.

Would a zero to the left of the 1 in 0.125 change the value of the decimal? The answer is *absolutely YES* because 0.0125 is $\frac{125}{10000}$ and can't be reduced to $\frac{125}{1000}$.

**Question:**   Which of the following is the largest number: 0.12 or 0.0978?

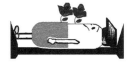

You might have selected 0.0978, and you might also have killed the patient!

The number 0.12 is also written $\frac{12}{100}$. The decimal 0.0978 is equal to $\frac{978}{10000}$. So far, it might be hard to tell which is larger, because these two fractions are very different in appearance.

Gee, I wonder if there is a way to make the fractions look similar. What if we gave $\frac{12}{100}$ and $\frac{978}{10000}$ common denominators?

The common denominator would be 10,000. Thus, $\frac{12}{100}$ would become $\frac{1200}{10000}$, which is larger than $\frac{978}{10000}$. This means 0.12 is larger than 0.0978.

## Converting Common Fractions to Decimals

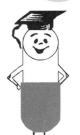

*To convert fractions to decimals, divide the numerator by the denominator.*

**Question:** If you have the fraction ½, how do you convert it to a decimal fraction?

***All right, I know you can do this with a calculator, but to better understand the process, please work it below.***

**Solution:** Take the numerator (1) and divide it by the denominator (2). Your answer is 0.5 or $\frac{5}{10}$, read *five-tenths.*

**Question:** Now that you think you have mastered the process, please show me the decimal fraction value for $\frac{3}{8}$.

**Solution:** Divide the numerator (3) by the denominator (8), which will give you the decimal fraction 0.375; this is equal to $\frac{375}{1000}$ and is read *three hundred and seventy-five thousandths.*

**Question:** Let's try a tougher one. Write the decimal fraction for $132\frac{3}{4}$.

**Solution:** Divide 3 by 4, which gives you the decimal 0.75, and then place the whole number 132 to the left of the decimal point. Our new decimal fraction is 132.75 and is read *one hundred and thirty-two and seventy-five hundredths.*

## Converting Decimals to Common Fractions

*To convert decimals to common fractions, simply express the decimal as a fraction and reduce it to the lowest terms.*

**Question:** Convert 0.25 to a common fraction.

**Solution:** 0.25 is the same as $\frac{25}{100}$. Reduce this number to the lowest terms, and you will have the common fraction $\frac{1}{4}$.

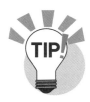

*To check your answer of $\frac{1}{4}$, divide 1 by 4 and you will have the decimal fraction 0.25.*

**Question:** Convert 0.125 to a common fraction.

**Solution:** 0.125 expressed as a common fraction is $\frac{125}{1000}$ and can be reduced to $\frac{1}{8}$. Check your answer by dividing 1 by 8.

**Question:**    Express 111.004 as a common fraction.

**Solution:**    0.004 expressed as a common fraction is $\frac{4}{1000}$ and can be reduced to $\frac{1}{250}$. The reduced common fraction is $111\frac{1}{250}$.

## Adding and Subtracting Decimal Fractions

*When adding and subtracting decimal fractions, make sure the decimal points line up vertically. Add additional zeros to the right and left of the numbers to make all numbers of equal length and to avoid errors.*

**Example:**    $0.135 + 1.21 + 153.1 = ?$

**Solution:**

$$
\begin{array}{r}
\mathbf{00}0.135 \\
\mathbf{00}1.21\mathbf{0} \\
+\,153.10\mathbf{0} \\
\hline
\text{answer } 154.445
\end{array}
$$

**Question:**    Solve the following: $14.012 - 3.11 = ?$

**Solution:**

$$
\begin{array}{r}
14.012 \\
-\,\mathbf{0}3.11\mathbf{0} \\
\hline
\text{answer } 10.902
\end{array}
$$

## Multiplying Decimal Fractions

*Count the total number of decimal places in the numbers multiplied and place the decimal point in the product (answer) to the left of the number of places counted (count from the right).*

**Confused? Let's look at an example to better explain this procedure.**

**Example:**    Solve the following: $216.3 \times 8.25 = ?$

$$
\begin{array}{rl}
216.3 & \text{(one decimal place)} \\
\times\,8.25 & \text{(two decimal places)} \\
\hline
1784475. &
\end{array}
$$

*Why is this answer incorrect?*

**Answer:**    Because the decimal point has not been correctly placed.

*The correct answer is 1784.475 because there was a total of three decimal places in the two numbers multiplied and it is necessary to place the decimal point in the answer three places from the right.*

## Dividing Decimal Fractions

*When dividing decimals, move the decimal points in the divisor and the dividend to the right to create "whole" numbers. Make sure you move each decimal point an EQUAL number of places and add zeros if necessary.*

**Example:**    $3.5 \div 1.5 = ?$
$35 \div 15 = 2.333333$ (round off to two decimal places) $= 2.33$

Here, both decimal points were moved one place to the right, but what would you do with the following example?

**Example:**    $6.85 \div 4.6 = ?$
$685 \div 460 = 1.48913$ (round off to two decimal places) $= 1.49$

*Since the decimal point in 6.85 was moved two places to the right, it was necessary to add an extra zero to 4.6 so that its decimal point could also be moved two places.*

*Have you noticed that I do not put a decimal point to the right of whole numbers? This is appropriate because there is no need to place it there.*

**Question:**    Please divide the following numbers and round off your answer.
$22.87 \div 0.107 = ?$

**Solution:**    $22.87 \div 0.107 = ?$
$22870 \div 107 = 213.73831 = 213.74 = 214$

*I have my own rule for rounding off numbers that will keep your answers within approximately 1% of the correct answer. In the first two examples I rounded off to two decimal places. I do this whenever there is only one whole number to the left of the decimal point. If you have two whole numbers, then round off to one decimal place. And in the last question, we had three whole numbers, so I dropped all the decimal places.*

*There are some areas of pharmacy practice (though rare) that may require you to be more accurate.*

## Multiplying and Dividing Decimals by Powers of Ten

*When multiplying decimals by powers of ten, move the decimal point as many places to the RIGHT as there are zeros in the multiplier. When dividing by powers of ten, move the decimal point to the LEFT as many places as there are zeros in the divisor.*

**Examples:**   $4.83 \times 10 = ?$ (move the decimal point one place to the right) $= 48.3$

$0.035 \times 1000 = ?$ (move the decimal point three places to the right) $= 35$

*This rule is especially good for estimating your answers. Example: $2.1 \times 300 = ?$ In this example, move the decimal point two places to the right and multiply by three (i.e., $2.1 \times 300 = 210 \times 3 = 630$). This style of estimation takes some practice, but it is a great skill to master and is worth the extra effort.*

**Examples:**   $72.62 \div 10 = ?$ (move the decimal point one place to the left) $= 7.262$

$367.3 \div 100 = ?$ (move the decimal point two places to the left) $= 3.673$

**Question:**   I bought a 5.5-pound roast, and you laughed and said you had a bull that weighed 4000 times that amount. Estimate the weight of the animal—is there a possibility you might be exaggerating?

**Solution:**   $5.5 \times 4000 = ?$ Because there are three zeros, move the decimal point three places to the right and multiply by four. That is, $5500 \times 4 = 22{,}000$ pounds

*I think you were "shooting the bull"! (no pun intended)*

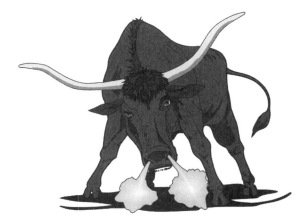

## PRACTICE

**13.** Add the following decimal fractions:

   (a) 15        +     1.5      +     0.15     +     150   =   **?**

   (b) 3.25      +     13.091   +     0.18   =   **?**

   (c) 0.38      +     0.097   +     0.0062   =   **?**

   (d) 22.0008  +     8.022   =   **?**

**14.** Subtract the following decimal fractions:

   (a) 32      –    1.0009   =   **?**     (c) 491.08   –   321.008   =   **?**

   (b) 2.52    –    0.333   =   **?**     (d) 0.0678   –   0.00678   =   **?**

**15.** Divide the following decimal fractions:

   (a) 23.8   ÷   0.294   =   **?**     (c) 341.44  ÷   0.37   =   **?**

   (b) 0.91   ÷   8.27   =   **?**     (d) 68.2   ÷   2000   =   **?**
                                            ***(try to guess this one before working it)***

**16.** Multiply the following decimal fractions:

   (a) 0.003  ×   0.09   =   **?**     (c) 100.25  ×   100.35   =   **?**

   (b) 54.5   ×   25.12   =   **?**     (d) 1336   ×   10,000   =   **?**
                                            ***(try to guess this one before working it)***

*I have an idea. Why don't we put the entire chapter together and create some stress, I mean some confidence!*

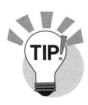

*Make sure all numbers are in the same system before calculating.*

**17.** Solve the following and reduce to lowest terms:

   (a) XXIV     ×      3.25   =   **?**

   (b) 26.23    ×     $6\frac{7}{12}$   =   **?**

   (c) LXVI    +     41.9   +   $333\frac{1}{2}$   =   **?**

   (d) cxiiiss  times    $8\frac{3}{8}$   =   **?**

    (e)   LXVII     –     XLII    =    **?**        (give answer in Roman numerals)

    (f)   17.1     $\div$     $4\frac{3}{8}$    =    **?**

    (g)   $3\frac{3}{4}$     $\div$     3.089    =    **?**

    (h)   5.029     $\times$     $19\frac{7}{8}$    =    **?**

    (i)   $13\frac{1}{4}$     $\div$     $\frac{1}{50}$    =    **?**        (give answer in Roman numerals)

    (j)   6.25     $\times$     $\frac{5}{8}$    =    **?**        (give answer as a decimal fraction)

    (k)   $\frac{1}{4}$     $\times$     **?**    =    48

    (l)   $(0.5 \div 2)$     $\times$     **?**    =    2

    (m)   $\left(\frac{1}{12} \div \frac{1}{15}\right)$     $\times$     30    =    **?**

**18.** A bottle of olive oil contains 96 teaspoons of oil. If you put an average of $4\frac{4}{5}$ teaspoons of olive oil on a salad, how many salads can you prepare?

**19.** If you prepare $8\frac{1}{2}$ meals from a box of oatmeal that weighs XXXII ounces, how many ounces of oatmeal are in each meal (expressed as a decimal fraction)?

**20.** If the average pharmacy technician can prepare CIX prescriptions per day, how many technicians are required to prepare MDCXXXV prescriptions?

**21.** A pharmacy technician has 100 grams of drug A on hand. How much will remain if she fills three prescriptions for capsules containing the following:

Rx 1        #30 capsules, each containing $1\frac{1}{4}$ grams of drug A
Rx 2        #15 capsules, each containing 2.75 grams of drug A
Rx 3        #10 capsules, each containing iss grams of drug A

**22.** How many capsules containing $1\frac{3}{4}$ grams of drug A can be prepared from the remainder of drug A in Question 21 (given as a decimal fraction)?

**23.** If a combination cold capsule contains 32.5 milligrams of drug B, $15\frac{3}{8}$ milligrams of drug C, 75.5 milligrams of drug D, and $118\frac{1}{8}$ milligrams of drug E, how many total milligrams (expressed in Roman numerals) are contained in each capsule?

**24.** How many 0.00055-gram doses can be made from $\frac{3}{4}$ gram of a drug?

**25.** If 1 kilogram of antiseptic powder costs $350, how much does 0.001 kilogram cost?

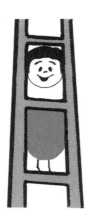

## ADVANCED PRACTICE QUESTIONS

*Each chapter will end with "Advanced Practice Questions." These are intended to challenge you and help develop your critical thinking skills. These questions will frequently require more than one step to solve. Please do not panic if you have difficulty solving these problems. Future chapters will provide you with the additional skills necessary to answer them easily. Good luck!*

**26.** A pharmacist purchases 4 ounces of codeine sulfate and dispenses the following quantities in preparing three prescriptions:

$\frac{1}{8}$ ounce

$\frac{1}{4}$ ounce

$1\frac{1}{2}$ ounces

How many ounces of codeine sulfate remain after preparing the prescriptions?

**27.** A set of alkaline batteries lasts 5 hours and 30 minutes in my daughter's CD player. For how many hours will the CD player run on 20 sets of batteries?

(Answer in Roman numerals.)

**28.** A recipe for 60,000 tablets calls for 45 grams of a specific drug. How many grams will each tablet contain?

**29.** In my daughter's chemistry laboratory, she had 58 milliliters of a chemical. On three occasions she withdrew the following quantities using a pipette:

First occasion     14        milliliters
Second occasion    4.75      milliliters
Third occasion     $3\frac{3}{4}$     milliliters

How many milliliters remained in the bottle after the third withdrawal of the chemical?

**30.** Using a suppository mold, I made a dozen suppositories from 1.5 grams of a drug. How much of the drug was contained in each suppository? (Give your answer as a common fraction.)

**31.** A pharmacy technician at Foothills Pharmacy filled two dozen small bottles with a concentrated antiseptic solution. How many ounces of the solution were needed in total if each bottle contained $2\frac{2}{3}$ ounces?

**32.** Nadia receives $1\frac{1}{2}$ teaspoons (7.5 milliliters) of an antibiotic three times a day. How many full days does the medication last if the pharmacy dispensed two 200-milliliter bottles of the medication?

**33.** Hadley receives $1\frac{2}{3}$ ounces of a medication daily for 7 days in divided doses. She then receives half of the initial daily dose for another week. How many ounces did the pharmacist need to dispense to provide the 2 weeks of therapy?

**34.** Fluticasone propionate inhalation aerosol is available in various strengths. What would be the strength of a canister that is $\frac{1}{5}$ the potency of the 220-microgram per actuation dosage form?

**35.** Tres-Lyte supplement contains $\frac{16}{100}$ gram of sodium, $\frac{28}{100}$ gram of potassium, and $\frac{25}{100}$ gram of phosphorus per packet. How many total grams of these electrolytes are in a 100-packet box? (Note: I like this supplement so much that I plan to ask about it again, maybe in the next chapter and the next one too.)

*The answers to all problems can be found in the **Answer Key** beginning on page 253.*

*Now, if you understand Chapter 1 really well, let's go figure out what these grams, milligrams, kilograms, and Cheerios® are all about.*

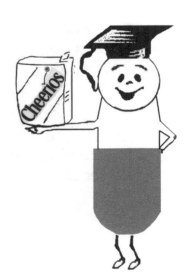

# Systems of Measurement

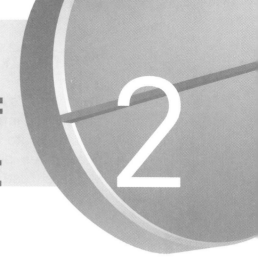

2

In Chapter 1, we reviewed the fundamentals of mathematics that will be used throughout this textbook. Before we get into the "meat and potatoes" of pharmaceutical calculations, I want you to master one more foundational area: the systems of measurement.

In Chapter 1, we reviewed the fundamentals of mathematics that will be used throughout this textbook. Before we get into the "meat and potatoes" of pharmaceutical calculations, I want you to master one more foundational area: the systems of measurement.

Most textbooks focus on the three systems of measurement (metric, apothecary, and avoirdupois), but I will focus on the metric and only briefly mention the other two systems. My reasoning is that the metric system has been adopted and mandated in the United States and throughout the world as the standard for pharmaceutical and medical calculations.

In addition, the U.S. Pharmacopeial Convention, the National Association of Boards of Pharmacy, and other "standard-setting" organizations have embraced the metric system as the sole system of measurement. As a pharmacy technician, you need to master the metric system, but you should also know that there are other systems just in case they appear on a prescription or an old compounding formula.

The metric system has three primary units:
- ☐ the **meter,** which measures length,
- ☐ the **liter,** which is used for volume, and
- ☐ the **gram,** which measures weight.

## OBJECTIVES

Upon mastery of Chapter 2 you will be able to:

- Understand the guidelines for metric notation.
- Recognize the apothecary and avoirdupois systems of measurement.
- Perform basic math functions using the systems of measurement.
- Relate the metric system to "household" equivalents utilized by patients.

# Metric System

The metric system is a decimal system, meaning that each primary unit is subdivided into multiples of ten. In the metric system, prefixes for the primary units indicate what segment of the unit is being considered. There are more than 16 prefixes, but since I can't remember most of them, and more importantly you will rarely use the majority of them, I will focus on the following four:

*Here are*
       *the important ones !!!*

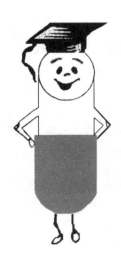

*kilo*   = 1000 or one thousand

*centi*  = $\frac{1}{100}$ or 0.01 or one hundredth

*milli*   = $\frac{1}{1000}$ or 0.001 or one thousandth

*micro* = $\frac{1}{1000000}$ or 0.000001 or one millionth

*So how do all these prefixes and primary units relate to pharmacy?*

**Here are metric measurements and abbreviations you will encounter frequently in everyday medical and pharmacy practice:**

| *LENGTH* | | | *WEIGHT* | | |
|---|---|---|---|---|---|
| meter | (m) | | gram | (g or Gm) | |
| centimeter | (cm) | $\frac{1}{100}$ of a meter | milligram | (mg) | $\frac{1}{1000}$ of a gram |
| millimeter | (mm) | $\frac{1}{1000}$ of a meter | microgram | (mcg *or* μg) | $\frac{1}{1000000}$ of a gram |
| | | | kilogram | (kg *or* Kg) | 1000 grams |

*VOLUME*

liter       (l or L)

milliliter    (ml or mL) $\frac{1}{1000}$ of a liter

A cubic centimeter (cc) is sometimes used by practitioners to denote a milliliter.

# Guidelines for Metric Notation

1. **Always place the number before the abbreviation.**
   8 mL, not mL 8

2. **Place a zero to the left of the decimal when the decimal fraction is less than 1.**
   Digoxin 0.125 mg, not digoxin .125 mg. (The zero draws attention to the decimal and decreases the possibility of giving the wrong dose; in this case, 125 mg might be given if the decimal is not noticed.)

3. **Never place a zero to the right of the decimal place when you have a whole number.** A patient weighs 11 kg, not 11.0 kg. (The zero in this example may mask the decimal, and the weight might be read as 110 kg.)

4. **Always use decimals to represent fractions when using the metric system.**
   3.5 mg, not $3\frac{1}{2}$ mg.

5. **Avoid unnecessary zeros.**
   60.02000 g should be written 60.02 g because the last 3 zeros have no value. However, zeros *between* whole numbers are very important to interpret the numbers accurately.

6. **Always think carefully when converting from subunits.** When going from a smaller unit to a larger unit, make sure your number *decreases* proportionately. Example: Convert 5675 mg to grams.
   A gram is 1000 times larger than a milligram, so the number to the left of the primary unit must be divided by 1000. In this example, 5675 mg = 5.675 g.

7. **When converting from a larger unit to a smaller unit,** make sure your number *increases* proportionately.
   Example: Convert 72 kg to grams.
   A gram is 1000 times smaller than a kilogram, so the number to the left of the primary unit (i.e., gram) must be multiplied by 1000.
   In this example, 72 kg = 72,000 g.

8. **When multiplying metric values by multiples of ten,** move the decimal point one place to the *right* for each zero in the multiplier.
   10　×　84.67　=　846.7
   1000　×　0.325　=　325

9. **When dividing metric values by multiples of ten,** move the decimal point one place to the *left* for each zero in the divisor.
   74.67　÷　100　=　0.7467
   0.67　÷　1000　=　0.00067

10. **When in doubt, check it out!** Always check when clarification is needed.
    A one-decimal-place error in dosing can frequently be **fatal** to a patient, so be careful.

# PRACTICE

1. Convert the following metric units:

   (a)  25 kg        = ? g      answer ___25000___

   (b)  55 g         = ? mg     answer ___55,000___  55 x 1000

   (c)  72 mg        = ? mcg    answer ___72 x 1000 = 72000___

   (d)  105 L        = ? mL     answer ___105 x 105000___

   (e)  48 m         = ? cm     answer ___4800___  48 x 100

   (f)  1257 mm      = ? m      answer ___1.257___  1257 ÷ 1000

   (g)  387 cm       = ? mm     answer ___38700___  387 x 10

   (h)  43 mm        = ? cm     answer ___4.3___  43 ÷ 10

   (i)  982 mg       = ? g      answer ___0.982___  982 ÷ 1000

   (j)  3389 mg      = ? kg     answer ___0.003389___  3389 ÷ 1000000

   (k)  0.0765 mg    = ? mcg    answer ___76.5___  0.0765 x 1000

   (l)  0.00376 g    = ? µg     answer _____

   (m)  5786 mL      = ? L      answer _____

   (n)  0.0698 L     = ? mL     answer _____

   (o)  0.00997 kg   = ? mg     answer _____

   (p)  8,023,766 g  = ? kg     answer _____

   (q)  7569 mcg     = ? g      answer _____

   (r)  355.56 mL    = ? L      answer _____

   (s)  0.0298 m     = ? mm     answer _____

   (t)  0.002289 mL  = ? L      answer _____

   (u)  0.200897 kg  = ? mcg    answer _____

*The answers to all problems can be found in the **Answer Key** beginning on page 253.*

If you had problems with Question 1, you need to review the previous material before continuing. If you are ready, then let's crank it up a notch and try some of the dreaded "word problems" using the metric system.

The best way to answer the following questions is to convert everything to the same units.

**Example:**    1 kg    +    300 g    =    ?

**Solution:**    1000 g    +    300 g    =    1300 g    *or*    1 kg    +    0.3 kg    =    1.3 kg

# PRACTICE

**2.** Yesterday I bought three cantaloupes of various weights. One weighed 635 g, another weighed 0.58 kg, and the third weighed 428,970 mg. How many grams did all three cantaloupes weigh?

> *I like to convert all the units to whatever unit is asked for in the answer.*

**3.** Yesterday I also purchased a really big bunch of white grapes weighing a whopping 1.27 kg. When I arrived home, I was so bored that I decided to count each and every little grape. Guess what? There was a total of 429 grapes. How many grams did each grape weigh?

**4.** I was on a tear yesterday at the grocery store and also bought a pound of coffee. If a pound weighs 454 g, how many pots of coffee can be prepared if each pot requires 22,700 mg of ground coffee?

**5.** My daughter Angela loves cranberry juice, so I bought her a bottle containing 64 fluid ounces. I noticed that on the bottle, next to the 64 fl oz, there was also the number 1.89 L. Since you're the new resident expert on the metric system, I am sure you immediately recognized what the 1.89 L means, but could you tell me how many 210-mL glasses of juice Angela can get from the bottle?

**6.** The grocery store is only 2.6 kilometers from my home. How many meters would I travel in a round-trip to the store and back home?

**7.** Last summer I gained 8 pounds on vacation. How many kilograms was this if there are 454 grams per pound?

*(By now you are probably thinking I'm a geek and wouldn't have a weight problem if I'd "get a life" and quit counting grapes!)*

**8.** My wife, Patricia, cut her finger. I noticed that the bandage she used was 7.62 cm in length and that the box contained 100 bandages. If I got very bored and decided to place the 99 remaining bandages end to end, how many meters would they stretch?

***Now let's apply the metric system to pharmacy practice.***

**9.** A pharmacy technician weighs four partially full bottles of salicylic acid. How many grams of salicylic acid does she have if the bottles contain 378 g, 0.86 kg, 198,000 mg, and 38,000,000 mcg?

**10.** A formula for a bulk salicylic acid ointment requires 1.5 kg of salicylic acid. You have on hand only the amount calculated in question 9. How many additional milligrams of salicylic acid must you purchase?

**11.** How many 120-mL bottles can be filled from 3.84 L of a cough syrup?

**12.** A pharmacy buys 3 kg of flea powder and repackages it into powder "shaker" cans containing 90 g each. How many shakers can be completely filled with powder?

**13.** How many grams of thiamine HCl would be required to prepare 2500 capsules that each contain 750 mcg of thiamine HCl?

**14.** How many 30-mg codeine capsules can be prepared from 0.0009 kg of codeine?

**15.** If a vial contains 40 mg of tobramycin sulfate per milliliter, how many micrograms of tobramycin sulfate are in 0.1 mL from the vial?

**16.** How many millimeters tall is a patient who was measured at 178 cm?

*The answers to all problems can be found in the **Answer Key** beginning on page 253.*

# Apothecaries' System

At the beginning of this chapter, I mentioned that the metric system was the primary and most recommended system of measurement used today. The apothecaries' system is antiquated but still occasionally appears in pharmacy and medical practice. This system measures weights and volumes, but it does not have a measure of length.

Although I do not recommend that you spend a lot of time with this section, it would behoove you to at least be familiar with the apothecaries' system so that you can make conversions to the metric system whenever necessary.

The grain is the primary unit of weight in the apothecaries' system. The abbreviation for grain (gr) is frequently confused with the abbreviation for gram (g), but these weights are very different. The pound in this system is not the same as the 16-ounce pound you are familiar with in everyday life. This pound only has 12 ounces. The grain is the only weight in this system that you will see frequently in contemporary pharmacy practice. All of these weights are being replaced by the metric system's gram.

## APOTHECARIES' WEIGHTS

| 20 grains (gr) | = | 1 scruple | (℈) | | |
|---|---|---|---|---|---|
| 3 scruples | = | 1 dram | (Ʒ) | = | 60 grains |
| 8 drams | = | 1 ounce | (℥) | = | 480 grains |
| 12 ounces | = | 1 pound | (℔) | = | 5760 grains |

## APOTHECARIES' FLUID MEASURES

| 60 minims (♏) | = | 1 fluid dram | (fƷ) | | |
|---|---|---|---|---|---|
| 8 fluid drams | = | 1 fluid ounce | (f℥) | = | 480 minims |
| 16 fluid ounces | = | 1 pint | (pt.) | | |
| 2 pints | = | 1 quart | (qt.) | = | 32 fluid ounces |
| 4 quarts (8 pints) | = | 1 gallon | (gal.) | = | 128 fluid ounces |

Ounces, pints, quarts, and gallons are the measures of volume that most of you see in everyday life. They will eventually be replaced by the liter and milliliter of the metric system.

## PRACTICE

**17.** Convert the following:

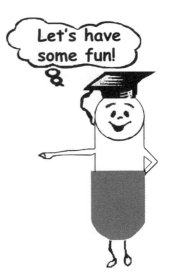

*Let's have some fun!*

(a)  5 quarts          =  _____ fluid ounces

(b)  3 gallons         =  _____ pints

(c)  498 pints         =  _____ gallons

(d)  322 fluid ounces  =  _____ quarts

(e)  960 minims        =  _____ fluid ounces

(f)  480 fluid drams   =  _____ fluid ounces

(g)  1/4 gallon        =  _____ pints

(h)  76 ounces         =  _____ grains

(i)  64 drams          =  _____ ounces

**18.** How many 4-fluid-ounce bottles can be filled from 2 gallons of elixir?

**19.** How many apothecaries' ounces of a drug would a patient receive in a week if she took 180 grains daily?

**20.** How many capsules containing $1\frac{3}{4}$ grains each of a drug can be prepared from $1\frac{3}{4}$ apothecaries' ounces of the drug?

*The answers to all problems can be found in the **Answer Key** beginning on page 253.*

## Avoirdupois System

The avoirdupois system is another antiquated system used only for measuring weight. Even though it too is being replaced by the metric system of weights, you will find that you are already familiar with its units even though you probably cannot pronounce the name of this system!

## AVOIRDUPOIS WEIGHTS

| 1 ounce (oz) | = | 437.5 grains (gr) | = | 28.4 g |
|---|---|---|---|---|
| 16 ounces | = | 1 pound (lb) | = | 7000 gr |

Did you notice what the apothecaries' and the avoirdupois systems of weights have in common? Of course you did. They both contain grains as the smallest unit.

Did you also notice that an ounce in one system has 437.5 gr and in the other has 480 gr? The ounce and the pound in the avoirdupois system of weights are the ones you use every day. The apothecaries' ounces and pounds are rarely (if ever) used, so don't spend your life worrying too much about that system of weights.

*Try a couple of problems!*

**21.** Convert the following:

(a) 168 lb = _____ oz     (d) 768 gr = _____ lb

(b) 137 oz = _____ lb     (e) 1276 gr = _____ oz

(c) 36 oz = _____ gr

**22.** A pharmacy technician found three containers of bismuth subnitrate powder containing: $1\frac{1}{8}$ lbs, 15 oz, and 3276 gr. How many total ounces of bismuth subnitrate powder did she find?

*Now let's figure out how to relate*
*all these crazy values to the metric system!*

# Common Conversion Factors

Several conversion factors will help you convert to the metric system when confronted with apothecaries' or avoirdupois values. I've rounded them off to keep you from going loony!

## METRIC CONVERSIONS

### *WEIGHT*

1 gram (g)      = 15.4 grains (gr)
1 gr            = 65 milligrams (mg) = 0.065 g
1 pound (lb)    = 454 g  = 0.454 kg
1 kilogram (kg) = 2.2 lb ($\frac{1000}{454}$ = 2.2)
1 ounce (oz)    = 28.4 g ($\frac{454}{16}$ = 28.4)

### *VOLUME*

1 fluid ounce = 30 milliliters (mL)
1 pint (pt)   = 16 fluid ounces
              = 480 mL
1 gallon      = 3840 mL

*Many times you will notice on a pint bottle that the volume is 473 mL. Why then would I tell you to use 480 mL? The reason is that manufacturers are using the exact equivalents and I'm rounding off. In reality, a fluid ounce contains 29.57 mL, and to calculate the volume of a pint you would multiply by 16, giving an answer of 473.12 mL per pint. So ask yourself, do you like my rounded-off numbers or the real numbers? Most pharmacies will use the rounded-off 480-mL conversion for a pint.*

## Household Equivalents

This last system of measurement has no real scientific basis. It was created to assist the patient with measuring while at home. Telling the average consumer to take "$\frac{1}{6}$ apothecaries' fluid ounce" of a cough syrup would be silly, and most patients wouldn't have a clue as to what you were saying. Instead, you can simply tell the patient to take 1 teaspoonful of the medication, and the patient will not only receive the correct dose but will smile and understand what you said.

This need for simple and accurate methods for measuring led to the evolution of household equivalents. There are many household equivalents (ex., dessert-spoonful, wine glass), but, as always, I will rescue you and only require you to learn the ones routinely seen in pharmacy practice.

1 teaspoonful (tsp)    =    5 milliliters (mL)
1 tablespoonful (tbsp) =    15 mL
1 fluid ounce (oz) (f℥) =    30 mL
1 pint (pt)            =    480 mL

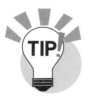

*Always make sure patients use measuring devices when they are directed to take a "teaspoon" or "tablespoon" dose. Why? Because teaspoons range in size from approximately 3 mL all the way to 7 mL, so there is great potential for error. Tablespoons can vary by almost 8 mL, which can also lead to significant problems in dosing. Due to the use of household equivalents, many liquid medications are prepared to contain a certain quantity of a drug per teaspoonful (5 mL). Some examples of this are amoxicillin 250 mg/5 mL and diphenhydramine 12.5 mg/5 mL. Physicians will tell the patient, in the case of the amoxicillin, to take "1 teaspoonful three times a day," and the patient will receive 250 mg in each dose. If a patient used a 3-mL teaspoon instead of a measuring device, he would receive only 150 mg of the amoxicillin instead of the recommended 250-mg dose. See how important you are?*

*Question:*    How many teaspoons are in a tablespoon?

*Answer:*    3    (3 × 5 mL = 15 mL)

*Question:*    How many tablespoons are in a pint?

*Answer:*    32    (480 ÷ 15 = 32)

# PRACTICE

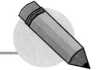

**23.** Convert the following:

(a)  4.5 teaspoons   =   _____ mL

(b)  325 lb          =   _____ kg

(c)  3000 gr         =   _____ g

(d)  289 kg          =   _____ lb

(e)  75 mL           =   _____ tsp

(f)  67 g            =   _____ gr

(g)  6.5 lb          =   _____ oz

(h)  118 mg          =   _____ gr

(i)  727 oz          =   _____ lb

(j)  1700 mL         =   _____ pt

(k)  43 gr           =   _____ mg

(l)  35 tbsp         =   _____ tsp

(m) 4.8 pints        =   _____ mL

(n)  3 fluid ounces  =   _____ tsp

(o)  64 fluid ounces =   _____ pints

(p)  111 kg          =   _____ lb

(q)  485 lb          =   _____ kg

(r)  4 quarts        =   _____ L

(s)  15,000 mL       =   _____ gallons

(t)  $5\frac{3}{4}$ lb          =   _____ g

(u)  2150 mL         =   _____ tbsp

(v)  $3\frac{1}{2}$ oz          =   _____ g

(w) 35 pints         =   _____ gallons

(x)  5 L             =   _____ pints

(y)  4000 mL         =   _____ fluid ounces

(z)  350 tsp         =   _____ L

*Now let's put it all together and do some pharmacy-related problems.*

24. A pharmacist dispensed four prescriptions for a narcotic in the following quantities: 18 gr, 2600 mg, 1.3 g, and ¼ avoirdupois ounce (oz).

(a) How many grains of narcotic were dispensed in all four prescriptions?

(b) How many milligrams of narcotic were dispensed in all four prescriptions?

(c) Prior to filling the four prescriptions, the pharmacy technician noted that there was ½ avoirdupois ounce (oz) of narcotic in stock. How many grams of narcotic remain after the four prescriptions have been filled?

25. A pharmacy technician prepared six prescriptions containing the following volumes: ⅛ gallon, ½ quart, ½ pint, 5 fl. ounces, 8 tbsp, and 15 tsp.

(a) How many teaspoons were dispensed in the six prescriptions?

(b) If the pharmacy technician started with a gallon of the substance, how many milliliters remain after filling the six prescriptions?

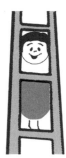

## ADVANCED PRACTICE QUESTIONS

26. How many milliliters will be left in a 4-liter bag of normal saline after the following quantities have been removed: 50 mL, 1 pint, 1 quart, and 0.75 L?

27. A patient receives 500 mcg of estradiol benzoate by injection every day for 3 weeks. How many grams of estradiol benzoate does the patient receive during the course of therapy?

28. One pint of an oil is used in manufacturing 1 million capsules. How many milliliters of oil are contained in each capsule?

**29.** Two kilograms of a drug are used to make 40,000 tablets.

(a) How many milligrams of the drug are in each tablet?

(b) How many grams would be required to make 60 tablets?

**30.** One pint of a cough syrup is dispensed to a patient who takes 1 tablespoonful of the syrup four times a day for a week. How many doses of the syrup remain in the original bottle after the full course of therapy?

**31.** Last month McKinney's Apothecary dispensed the following liquid medications: 1 gallon, 3 quarts, 7 pints, and three dozen 6-ounce bottles.

(a) In total, how many milliliters were dispensed?

(b) In total, how many gallons were dispensed?

**32.** Keylana's pediatrician recommended that she take 10 mg of acetaminophen per 1 kg of body weight (written 10 mg/kg) for her headache, but her mother (Angie) doesn't have a clue as to what Keylana weighs in the metric system. All Angie knows is that her little girl weighs 66 pounds.

(a) How many kilograms can you tell Angie her daughter weighs?

(b) How can you rewrite 10 mg/kg using pounds in the denominator instead of kg?

**33.** My grandson Beckett weighed a whopping 6 lb 15 oz when he was born.

(a) Express Beckett's birth weight in ounces.

(b) Express his birth weight in kilograms.

**34.** A bottle of nitroglycerin contains 25 tablets, each containing $\frac{1}{150}$ gr of nitroglycerin.

(a) How many milligrams of nitroglycerin are contained in each tablet?

(b) How many grams of nitroglycerin are in a bottle?

**35.** Question 35 in Chapter 1 discussed Tres-Lyte supplement, which contains $\frac{16}{100}$ g sodium, $\frac{28}{100}$ g potassium, and $\frac{25}{100}$ g phosphorus per packet. An entire box of the supplement contains 100 packets.

(a) How many milligrams of electrolytes are contained in 10 packets?

(b) How many micrograms of phosphorus are in an entire box of packets?

*The answers to all problems can be found in the **Answer Key** beginning on page 253.*

*If you have mastered the basics of pharmacy calculations, it is time to move to Chapter 3, the meat and taters of this book!*

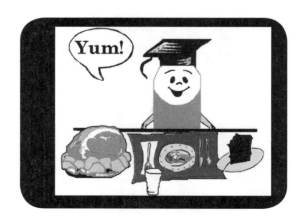

# Ratios and Proportions

In my opinion, Chapter 3 is the key to understanding how to perform almost every type of math problem you will encounter both in pharmacy practice and in everyday life. Your success in future chapters will hinge on how well you master this section. Calculations involving "drip rates," "milliequivalents," "percentages," and even "reducing and enlarging formulas" will be done by the exact same process.

As I mentioned in the preface, you do not need to know a lot of fancy math procedures to be successful with most medical and pharmaceutical calculations. This is easy material, but we will spend much more time than other textbooks do on ratios and proportions because I want you to really know this concept inside and out. By doing so, you will find that pharmacy calculations are, as they say back home, a "piece of cake"!

Back in Chapter 1, we discussed common fractions and decimals. Hopefully, you remember that the fraction $\frac{1}{2}$ is equal to 0.5, but did you know that this fraction can also be expressed as a percentage and as a ratio? In this chapter, we will focus on ratios. Later in the book I will cover percentages.

## OBJECTIVES

Upon mastery of Chapter 3 you will be able to:

- Express common and decimal fractions as ratios.
- Have an understanding of the process of ratio and proportion.
- Solve problems using the process of ratio and proportion.

*So it's off to the "ratio and proportion" races!*

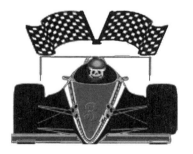

You know that 0.5 is equal to $\frac{5}{10}$ and also that $\frac{5}{10}$ can be reduced all the way down to $\frac{1}{2}$ by simply dividing the numerator and denominator by the number 5. These two fractions ($\frac{1}{2}$ and $\frac{5}{10}$) are exactly equal in value, with $\frac{1}{2}$ reduced to lowest terms.

**Question:** Are the fractions $\frac{3}{6}$, $\frac{4}{8}$, and $\frac{13}{26}$ also equal in value to $\frac{1}{2}$?

**Answer:** Yes, they are all equal. As an example, pull out your trusty calculator, and let's take a look at $\frac{13}{26}$, which is the toughest one of them. Divide 13 by 26, and your answer should be 0.5 (if it isn't, you need to buy another calculator!). Try this same process with the other fractions, and you will continue to get 0.5 as an answer.

**Question:** What fraction of apples would be eaten if you bought a dozen and ate 6?

**Answer:** The answer is that $\frac{6}{12}$ of the apples have been eaten. If you are really on a roll, you probably said that $\frac{1}{2}$ have been consumed. You may even have said that 0.5 of the apples have been eaten.

**Question:** What fraction of oranges would be still good if you started with 16 oranges and 12 of them rotted before you could eat them?

**Answer:** In this case, we would have $\frac{4}{16}$ of the oranges remaining. This can be reduced to $\frac{1}{4}$ by simply dividing the numerator and the denominator by the common number 4. This means that $\frac{4}{16}$ is equal to $\frac{1}{4}$, which is also equal to 0.25.

*The fraction of oranges that rotted is $\frac{12}{16}$, or $\frac{3}{4}$, or 0.75.*

## So What Is a Ratio?

Ratios are just a way of expressing the relationship of one quantity to another. When writing a ratio, you usually put a colon (:) between the numbers. Actually, a ratio is the same as a fraction, a percent, and even a decimal fraction.

I will not use ratios written with a colon very often in this text, but it is beneficial to have an understanding of the concept, because you will sometimes encounter ratios written that way in practice. We will discuss ratios in more depth in future chapters.

In most of the cases you will experience in pharmacy, the ratio indicates how much of a drug is in a solution.

**Example:** Epinephrine 1:1000 solution

The ratio 1:1000 indicates the amount of drug to the amount of total solution. This example means there is 1 part of epinephrine in 1000 parts of solution.

> The 1:1000 ratio can also be written as $\frac{1}{1000}$ or as 0.001.

**Example:** In the earlier question concerning apples, the ratio of eaten to total apples is 6:12 or 1:2 (when reduced). Do not get all caught up in this. I will usually write the 1:2 ratio as a fraction ($\frac{1}{2}$) and proceed from there.

**Question:** In the orange example, what is the ratio of edible oranges to total oranges?

**Answer:** 4:16, which is also the same as $\frac{4}{16}$ or $\frac{1}{4}$ or 1:4

*Now let's do something useful with all of these fractions!*

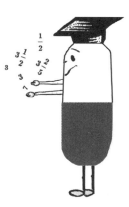

# Proportion

A proportion is the expression of the equality of two ratios or fractions to each other. For just a minute, I want you to think back to your pre-algebra coursework, when you learned all that stuff about (A/B = C/D). Does that bring back bad memories? We are not going to venture beyond this simple equation for your sake and for mine, but it is important for you to understand the concept.

The equation (A/B = C/D) is actually a proportion in which two equal fractions are put side by side. Let's set up a proportion based on our earlier discussion in this chapter by putting two equal fractions in a proportional equation. In the "apple" example, we said that $\frac{6}{12}$ was equal to $\frac{1}{2}$. To prepare a proportion, we simply put these fractions equal to each other, just like this: ($\frac{1}{2} = \frac{6}{12}$). This is the same as (A/B = C/D).

**So what?** Well, if in the "apple" example I had said only that you had 12 apples and ate $\frac{1}{2}$ of them, could you have told me how many were eaten? I bet you knew the answer was 6 without even solving it on paper. **Am I correct?** You actually performed a ratio and proportion problem in your cute little head and probably didn't know the process was taking place.

**Try another one.** If you have 24 eggs and break $\frac{1}{4}$ of them, how many eggs did you break? There is a good chance that you said 6 without thinking much about it. Or possibly you multiplied 24 times $\frac{1}{4}$ to get your answer: $24 \times \frac{1}{4} = 6$.

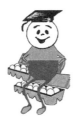

**The process really doesn't get much harder, so stay focused on what is happening.**

I want you to take a minute to solve the same problem by the process of ratio and proportion: (A/B = C/D) → 1/4 = C/24. OOPS! I'm missing a number over 24. We already know that the "C" is equal to "6," making the equation $\frac{1}{4} = \frac{6}{24}$, and we know that both fractions are equal, but what if the numbers were more complicated?

The overall process is very simple, but I believe it is best to learn with easy numbers and then advance to more complex ones. By remembering easy-to-understand examples like those discussed so far, you will be able to go back to those examples if you become confused.

You probably remember your teachers telling you "If you have the equation A/B = C/D and you know three of the numbers, you can solve for the missing fourth number." The method most people use (and the only one I will use) is cross multiplication. Simply multiply numerators by denominators and solve for the missing number.

*I like to use a question mark (?) for the "unknown" when solving ratio and proportion problems. Most people use an X, but I like the ?, because we will not confuse this sign with the "times" or "multiplying" symbol, "×."*

Now let's cross multiply and solve for an unknown.

**Example:**    Using the previous "egg" question, solve for (**?**):

$\frac{1}{4} = \frac{?}{24}$

**Step 1.** Multiply numerators by denominators (1 × 24) and (4 × **?**) and put them equal to each other.

(1 × 24)   =   (4 × **?**)

or

(1) (24)   =   (4) (**?**)

*I like to solve these problems with this format.*

**Step 2.** Now solve for (**?**):

(1) (24)   =   (4) (**?**)   *(Multiply the 1 by 24 to get 24.)*

24          =   (4) (**?**)

$\frac{24}{4}$          =   ?

6          =   ?

*This step is where many people make mistakes. You already knew that $\frac{1}{4}$ of 24 was 6, but now you know how to get there.*

*Now you try one.*

**Question:**   If a book has 68 pages, how many pages would there be in 30 of those books?

**Solution:**   **Step 1.** Set these two fractions equal to each other.

1 **book**/68 **pages**    = 30 **books**/(**?**)

**Step 2.** *Cross multiply* numerators by denominators.

1 **book**/68 **pages**     = 30 **books**/(**?**)
(68 **pages**)(30 **books**) = (1 **book**) (**?**)
2040 **pages** (**books**)  = 1 **book** (**?**)

**Step 3.** Divide and solve for (**?**).

2040 **pages** (**books**)/1 **book** = **?**
2040 **pages**                  = **?**

*The "book" units cancel when you divide, giving an answer in "pages."*

*Please stop right here!*

*Before we go any further, I want to ask you a question, and I want you to be honest. Did you estimate the answer to the last question?*

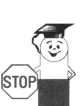

Your response is most likely *NO* if you are like the majority of my students and most practitioners. If you said *YES*, then you get a gold star, and I apologize for jumping on your case. As I mentioned earlier, you can avoid many "stupid" errors by simply estimating answers. In the last question, you could have easily said that 70 pages times 30 books equals 2100. (I know there were 68 pages, but you are just rounding off and estimating the correct answer.) What frequently happens in ratio and proportion problems is that people divide by the wrong number and get a ridiculous answer. In the last example, if you divided 68 by 30 you would get an answer of 2.27 pages. Does that make a lot of sense?

For the record, I would include 2.27 as a choice in a multiple-choice question to catch the "meatheads" who do not think and just start working problems without estimating.

Please take my word that you will be a better pharmacy technician or any other type of professional if you think a little before you act. This estimation process takes practice, but it should only take about 3–5 seconds per problem and is well worth the time and effort.

*OK, OK, enough lecturing. Let's get back to work!*

**Question:**    If 12 fishing hooks cost $1.25, how much will 20 hooks cost?

**Solution:**

| | | |
|---|---|---|
| 12 hooks/$1.25 = 20 hooks/? | *(set up proportion)* |
| (12 hooks) (**?**)  = ($1.25) (20 hooks) | *(cross multiply)* |
| 12 hooks (**?**)    = $25 hooks | |
| ?                   = $25 hooks/12 hooks | *(solve for ?)* |
| ?                   = $2.08 | |

*("Hooks" cancels when you divide, leaving your answer in dollars.)*

*I would estimate before solving this problem that since 12 hooks cost $1.25, 24 would cost about $2.50. (Since you want the price of 20 hooks, the answer will be less than $2.50.)*

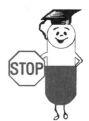

**Please stop again !!!**

All right, I've got one more question for you.

**Are you looking at the answers before working the questions or just skipping the "easy" stuff?**

Please work every problem in this book so that you get the full benefit. P.S. I'm sorry for jumping on your case if you are in the 5% of people who work in a methodical manner.

**Now let's have some fun!**

# PRACTICE

*Please work all problems in your book before checking answers.*

1.  Solve for the equivalent fractions, decimals, and ratio forms of the following numbers and reduce to lowest terms when necessary.

|     | **Fraction** | **Decimal** | **Ratio** |
|-----|--------------|-------------|-----------|
| (a) | $\frac{4}{12}$   | _____ | _____ |
| (b) | $\frac{20}{210}$ | _____ | _____ |
| (c) | $\frac{38}{218}$ | _____ | _____ |

|     |            |            |            |
|-----|------------|------------|------------|
| (d) | _____ | 0.6        | _____ |
| (e) | _____ | 0.005      | _____ |
| (f) | _____ | 0.44       | _____ |
| (g) | _____ | _____ | 3:15       |
| (h) | _____ | _____ | 30:600     |
| (i) | _____ | _____ | 600:2400   |

**2.** How many calories are in a 19-ounce box of Frosted Mini-Wheats® if there are 200 calories per serving? (A serving is 2.1 ounces.)

**3.** How many shampoos can I get out of a 750-mL bottle of Pert Plus® shampoo if I use approximately 1 teaspoonful of this product per shampoo?

*An advantage of being bald like me is that you don't need much shampoo!*

**4.** My daughter Kim teaches. She notes that the average student uses 75 sheets of paper every week.

    (a) How many sheets will a student use in a 42-week school year?

    (b) How many sheets will a class of 26 students use in a week?

**5.** A Diet Sprite® contains 2.92 mg of sodium per fluid ounce. How many grams of sodium are contained in a 12-ounce can?

*I'm trying to trick you with this question. See if you can beat me on this one.*

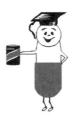

6.  My son Bill recently went to Central America for his honeymoon. While on this trip, he wanted to purchase his "honey" a gold bracelet that cost 480,000 *rumples*. (I really don't remember the correct currency name, but *rumples* sounds good enough for this question.) How much, in American currency, did the bracelet cost? *(1500 rumples = $1)*

7.  My baby daughter Abby goes through an average of one Pampers® diaper every 2 hours. How many diapers will we need to buy for a two-week vacation?

    *(It is difficult to relax on a vacation and change that many diapers!)*

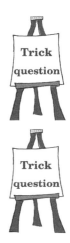

8.  If your car gets 18 miles per gallon of gasoline, how many pints of gas will you need to take a 698-mile trip?

9.  Coppertone Sport® Ultra Sweatproof SPF 15 dry lotion contains 1.2 mg of octylmethoxycinnamate per fluid ounce. How many micrograms of this chemical are in $\frac{1}{2}$ pint of the sunblock lotion?

10. If you could fill one prescription every 135 seconds, how many prescriptions could you fill every hour?

    *(Assuming no phone interruptions, lunch or bathroom breaks, or whiny patients!)*

11. A manufacturer wants to prepare 500,000 diazepam tablets, each containing 5 mg of diazepam. How many kilograms of diazepam will be required to prepare this batch?

12. If a drug contains 25 mg per tablespoon of an expectorant, how much expectorant is in a quart of this medication?

**13.** How much would 3 lb of sulfur cost if you purchased 182 lb of sulfur for $2134?

**14.** An antiflatulent medication contains 20 mg of simethicone per infant dose of 0.3 mL. How many grams of simethicone are contained in a 1-fluid-ounce bottle of the medication?

**15.** The average aspirin tablet contains 5 grains of acetylsalicylic acid (ASA). How many grams of ASA are in a 250-tablet bottle of aspirin?

**16.** A pharmacy technician prepared a large batch of zinc oxide ointment containing 10 grams of zinc oxide in every 100 grams of ointment. How much ointment was prepared if the technician used $\frac{3}{8}$ lb of zinc oxide?

**17.** A patient weighs 186 pounds, and the dosing schedule for a medication is given for weight measured in kilograms. How many kilograms does the patient weigh?

**18.** If an alprazolam tablet contains 0.25 mg of active ingredient, how many grains of alprazolam are contained in a 100-tablet bottle?

**19.** A pint of cough medicine contains 960 mg of an antitussive medication. How many grams of the medication are in a 2-teaspoonful dose?

20. How many milligrams of nitroglycerin are contained in 30 tablets that each contain $\frac{1}{150}$ gr of nitroglycerin?

21. If a patient receives 1.4 mL of 5% dextrose intravenous solution per minute, how many liters of solution does the patient receive in a day?

22. An injectable product contains 750 mcg of the active ingredient per vial. How many vials are needed to provide a 15-mg dose?

23. If a green soap tincture costs $32.00 per gallon, how much does a liter of the tincture cost?

24. A pharmacy technician prepares 3 liters of syrup using 5 lb of sugar. How many grams of sugar are in a teaspoonful of the syrup?

25. If 2 grains of phenobarbital are divided into 90 capsules, how many micrograms of phenobarbital are in each capsule?

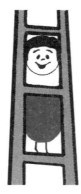

## ADVANCED PRACTICE QUESTIONS

26. A drug suspension costs $128.31 per pint. What would a week's supply of the suspension cost if a patient received 1 teaspoonful three times a day?

27. How many milligrams of nitroglycerin are in 60 tablets if each tablet contains $\frac{1}{100}$ grain of nitroglycerin?

**28.** A pound of an ointment costs $83.76. How much does it cost to fill a 3-ounce tube?

**29.** Each fluid ounce of an elixir contains 50 mg of codeine. How many grains of codeine are in $\frac{1}{2}$ fluid ounce of the elixir?

**30.** How many 2-mg tablets contain $\frac{3}{4}$ grain of a drug?

**31.** You need 0.5 gram of hydrocortisone to prepare a prescription. How many 20-mg hydrocortisone tablets are needed to supply the quantity of the drug required?

**32.** A patient is to receive 50 mg of amoxicillin orally. This drug is available in a strength of 125 mg per teaspoonful. How many milliliters of the drug provide the patient's appropriate dose?

**33.** A patient is to receive an IV solution at the rate of 200 milliliters per hour. How many 1-liter bags of the solution will the patient need each day?

**34.** A 2-mL vial of tobramycin sulfate contains 80 mg of the drug. How many milliliters of the injection should be administered to obtain 0.01 gram of tobramycin sulfate?

**35.** An intravenous set delivers 15 drops for every milliliter. How many drops are in $\frac{1}{2}$ liter of the intravenous solution?

**36.** Please look back at that dreaded question 35 in Chapter 1.

(a) What is the ratio of sodium to all electrolytes in a packet of Tres-Lyte supplement?

(b) What is the ratio of potassium to phosphorus in a packet?

**37.** Hydrocodone bitartrate and acetaminophen tablets USP are supplied in a 7.5 mg hydrocodone/650 mg acetaminophen strength and are available as scored tablets.

(a) Express this strength as a ratio of hydrocodone to acetaminophen.

(b) How many grams of hydrocodone does a patient receive in a $\frac{1}{2}$ tablet dose?

**38.** A 25-mcg liothyronine tablet is equivalent to approximately 1 gr of desiccated thyroid or thyroglobulin and 0.1 mg of L-thyroxine.

(a) How many equivalent micrograms of L-thyroxine would a patient receive in two weeks if the patient took one 25-mcg liothyronine tablet daily?

(b) How many equivalent grams of desiccated thyroid would be contained in a 100-tablet bottle of 25-mcg liothyronine?

**39.** Carbidopa and levodopa is a combination product for the treatment of Parkinson's disease and syndrome. One of the strengths available is 25 mg/100 mg, which contains 25 mg of carbidopa and 100 mg of levodopa and is supplied in unit dose packages of 100.

    (a) How many grams of carbidopa would a patient receive if that patient took 90 tablets?

    (b) How many micrograms of levodopa would a patient receive by taking $\frac{1}{2}$ tablet daily for a week?

**40.** According to research, there was no evidence of impaired fertility when dipyridamole was administered to male and female rats at oral doses of up to 500 mg/kg/day.

    (a) How many total grams of dipyridamole would have been given to a 260-gram rat receiving the maximum dose over a 30-day period?

    (b) Express this maximum daily dose in mg/lb/day.

*The answers to all problems can be found in the **Answer Key** beginning on page 253.*

# Interpreting Drug Orders and Calculating Doses

**4**

In Chapter 4, we will take all your skills from the first three chapters and apply them in calculating doses of medications. Before you start doing the math, you must first learn a few more foundational skills.

At the beginning of this chapter, you will learn how to interpret a written drug order. Later we will work some calculations related to drug orders. I have some great news for you. The math is exactly like the ratio and proportion questions you did in Chapter 3. I will just change the questions a little to relate more to individual patients.

The terms *dose* and *dosage* warrant clarification so that you know what I'm talking about.

A **dose** is the quantity of a drug taken by a patient. It may be expressed as a "daily" dose, a "single" dose, or even a "total" dose, which refers to all of the drug taken throughout therapy. A "daily" dose may be given once daily, which is a "single" daily dose, or it may be divided throughout the day, which would then be known as a "divided" dose.

***Example:*** If a physician orders 100 mg every morning, this would be a single dose. If the physician orders 100 mg in divided doses every 6 hours, you would give 25 mg every 6 hours (to total 100 mg/day).

Doses vary tremendously due to differences in drug potency, routes of administration, and the patient's age, weight, protein binding, and kidney and liver function. Many factors enter into establishing a correct dose, and many dispensing errors are related either to giving the wrong dose or to misinterpreting an order.

## OBJECTIVES

Upon mastery of Chapter 4 you will be able to:

- Write standard medical abbreviations.
- Read medical notations and determine a dosage regimen.
- Calculate appropriate doses for patients.
- Perform flow rate calculations.
- Solve for a dose using body surface area (BSA).
- Determine appropriate doses for chemotherapy using BSA.

As a pharmacy technician, you can contribute greatly to patient care by being able to calculate doses and read medication "orders." With these skills, you will eventually catch mistakes that have been overlooked by other health-care providers. So if you want to be the best technician in town, learn appropriate doses and dosage regimens and don't be afraid to speak up if you spot an error.

A **dosage regimen** refers to a schedule of medication administration. Here's a possible regimen you might encounter.

*Example:*    If a physician orders 250 mg every 6 hours, the *dose* is 250 mg, and the *dosage regimen* is "every 6 hours."

In many pharmacy calculation textbooks, you will encounter a truckload of rules for calculating doses. Names for some of these rules include Young's rule, Clark's rule, Fried's rule, and Cowling's rule. Unfortunately, these rules treat children and infants as just "little adults," with no consideration of any other physiological factors. Do not use them under any circumstances.

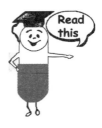

I have *never* seen anyone use those rules to dose. In every case you will encounter, appropriate doses will be specified by the manufacturer in the package inserts. Suitable doses can also be found in numerous references, such as the *Physicians' Desk Reference* (PDR) and *Drug Facts and Comparisons*. Doses are listed according to age and are given in milligrams or milliliters per kilogram or pound of body weight.

**All you need to know to calculate doses is our friend ratio and proportion.**

Before we start learning abbreviations, you need to know about one more thing—the drug order—which is the "bread and butter" of your job as a pharmacy technician.

*You are going to be mad at me now! Guess what?*

*Now you need to take a lot of time to memorize the following abbreviations, all of which you will encounter frequently in routine pharmacy practice.*

*Please do not continue before learning these abbreviations. (See the table in Chapter 13 for a list of potential problems associated with certain abbreviations.)*

# Common Medical Abbreviations

## FREQUENCY

| | | | | |
|---|---|---|---|---|
| a.c. | before meals | | p.c. | after meals |
| a.m. | morning | | h.s. | at bedtime |
| p.m. | afternoon or evening | | q.d. | once daily |
| ad. lib. | as desired | | stat | immediately |
| p.r.n. | as needed | | q.o.d. | every other day |
| b.i.d. | twice a day | | t.i.d. | three times a day |
| q.i.d. | four times a day | | min. | minute |
| h. or hr. | hour | | q.h. | every hour |
| q.2h | every 2 hours | | q.8h | every 8 hours |
| q.12h | every 12 hours | | u.d. | as directed |

## ROUTE

| | | | | |
|---|---|---|---|---|
| a.d. | right ear | | a.s. | left ear |
| a.u. | both ears | | IM | intramuscular |
| inj. | injection | | IV | intravenous |
| IVPB | intravenous piggyback | | IVP | intravenous push |
| o.d. | right eye | | o.u. | both eyes |
| o.s. or o.l. | left eye | | p.o. | by mouth |
| pr, p.r., PR | per rectum | | SL | sublingual |
| SC or SQ | subcutaneous | | ID | intradermal |

## DOSAGE FORMS

| | | | | |
|---|---|---|---|---|
| aq. | aqueous (water) | | cap | capsule |
| comp. | compound | | gtt. | drop |
| pulv | powder | | sol. | solution |
| supp. | suppository | | susp. | suspension |
| syr. | syrup | | tab | tablet |
| tinct or tr | tincture | | ung | ointment |

## MISCELLANEOUS

| | | | | |
|---|---|---|---|---|
| a | before | | p | after |
| c | with | | s | without |
| q | every | | ad | up to |
| a.a. | of each | | ante | before |
| DC, d/c, or disc. | discontinue | | dil. | dilute |
| disp. | dispense | | div. | divide |
| d.t.d. | give of such doses | | dx | diagnosis |
| et | and | | ft. | make |
| N/V | nausea and vomiting | | hx | history |
| q.s. | a sufficient quantity | | rt. | right |
| non rep. or N.R. | do not repeat | | GI | gastrointestinal |
| R/O | ruled out | | noct. | night |
| NPO | nothing by mouth | | Sig | write on label |
| SOB | shortness of breath | | BP | blood pressure |
| UTI | urinary tract infection | | M | mix |
| URI | upper respiratory infection | | HA | headache |

The **drug order** consists of seven parts that should always be present. Many state boards of pharmacy require additional information, but the following parts are the "biggies" you must know to fill a prescription correctly:

- Name of the patient to receive the medication.
- Name of the drug to be dispensed or administered.
- Dose of the drug.
- Route by which the drug is to be taken or administered.
- Dosage regimen by which the drug is to be taken or administered.
- Date (and time in institutional settings) when the order was written.
- Signature of the person writing the order or prescription.

*Prescriptions and drug orders differ in that drug orders are utilized in institutions and prescriptions are used in outpatient (community) settings. The legal requirements by which practitioners communicate medication requests vary with each of these methods.*

***Example:***    Prescription:
Ampicillin 250 mg caps.
Sig.    i cap. p.o. q.i.d.

"Sig." means to type on the label the following: Take 1 capsule by mouth 4 times a day.

***Example:***    Physician's drug order:
Demerol® 50 mg IM q.2-3h p.r.n. pain

For this order, the nurse would administer 50 mg of Demerol® intramuscularly every 2 to 3 hours as needed for pain.

***Question:***    Now write down what the following prescription means.
***(don't peek at the answer)***

Reglan 10 mg
i tab. p.o., q.i.d., a.c. and h.s.

***Answer:***    Take 1 tablet by mouth, four times a day, before meals and at bedtime.

## Body Surface Area (BSA)

One last topic in the area of dosing that you need to be familiar with is **body surface area,** also referred to as BSA. This procedure uses a patient's volume rather than the patient's weight. It is frequently used with patients receiving chemotherapy and sometimes with children. Body surface area is measured in square meters ($m^2$); most of the dosing we will see is in milligrams per square meter (mg/m²). These problems are also solved by ratio and proportion. Just substitute the appropriate BSA for weight in our equation.

But how do I solve for body surface area?

See the following nomograms for the determination of BSA. Please note that there is a nomogram for children (page 56) and one for adults (page 57). To solve for BSA, there are five steps.

**Step 1.** Make sure you are looking at the correct nomogram, i.e., adult or child.
**Step 2.** Place a dot on the patient's weight on the vertical line to the right.
**Step 3.** Place a dot on the patient's height on the vertical line to the left.
**Step 4.** Connect the dots by drawing a line with a straight edge.
**Step 5.** Read the patient's BSA, located on the center vertical line at the point where the line you drew in **Step 4** intersects it.

*Question:* What is the BSA for a child who is 32 inches tall and weighs 45 pounds?

*Answer:* Make sure you are using the *child* nomogram, and place dots on the 32-inch mark (left column) and on the 45-lb mark (right column). Connect the dots with a straight line. The BSA of 0.63 m² for this child is located on the center line.

*Question:* What is the BSA for a 52-year-old man who is 170 cm tall and weighs 70 kg?

*Answer:* Use the *adult* nomogram. The BSA for this patient is approximately 1.8 m².

*Question:* What would be the dose of a medication for the child in the first question if the medication was normally dosed at 50 mg/m²?

*Answer:* Solve by ratio and proportion: 50 **mg**/1 **m²** = **?**/0.63 **m²**
31.5 **mg** = **?** (the child's dose)

*Question:* What would be the dose in micrograms if the dose of a drug for the 52-year-old man in the second question was 0.04 mg/m²?

*Answer:* Change the dose to mcg at the beginning to make this easier: 40 mcg.
40 **mcg**/1 **m²** = **?**/1.8 **m²**
72 **mcg** = **?** (the patient's dose)

# Nomogram for Children
Determination of body surface from height and mass[1]

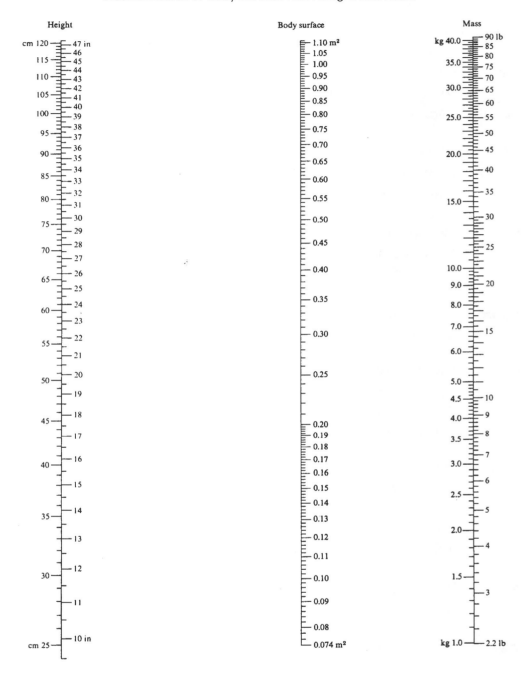

[1] From the formula of Du Bois and Du Bois, *Arch Intern Med*, 17, 863 (1916): $S = M^{0.425} \times H^{0.725} \times 71.84$, or $\log S = \log M \times 0.425 + \log H \times 0.725 + 1.8564$ ($S$ = body surface in cm², $M$ = mass in kg, $H$ = height in cm).

Source: C. Lentner, Ed., *Geigy Scientific Tables*, 8th ed, vol 1, Basel: Ciba-Geigy; 1981: 226–7.

# Nomogram for Adults
Determination of body surface from height and mass[1]

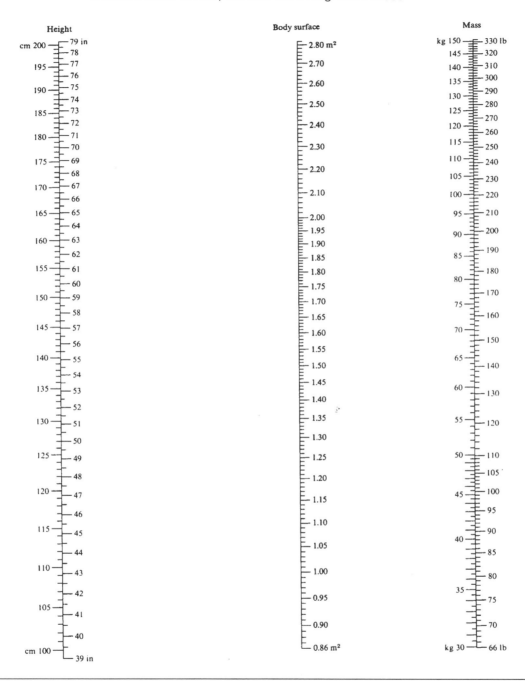

[1] From the formula of Du Bois and Du Bois, *Arch Intern Med,* 17, 863 (1916): $S = M^{0.425} \times H^{0.725} \times 71.84$, or
$\log S = \log M \times 0.425 + \log H \times 0.725 + 1.8564$ ($S$ = body surface in cm², $M$ = mass in kg, $H$ = height in cm).

Source: C. Lentner, Ed., *Geigy Scientific Tables,* 8th ed, vol 1, Basel: Ciba-Geigy; 1981: 226–7.

# Chemotherapy Dosing

In the last section, I mentioned that the body surface area (BSA) method of calculating doses is frequently used for cancer patients receiving chemotherapy. There are many safety considerations that must be taken into account in prescribing, compounding, and administering antineoplastic drugs. It is beyond the scope of this textbook to discuss these issues, but you need to be aware that specialized training is required for handling many chemotherapy products. Now let's solve for chemotherapy doses utilizing the body surface area method.

**Example:** Paclitaxel is an antineoplastic drug used to treat various carcinomas, including ovarian and breast cancer. How many milligrams of paclitaxel would a 42-year-old, 131-lb, 65-inch-tall female receive if the intravenous adult dose for breast carcinoma is 175 mg per square meter of body surface area repeated every twenty-one days?

**Solution:** Utilizing the nomogram for *adults*, the woman's BSA is approximately 1.65 m². Now plug in your numbers and perform a ratio and proportion calculation.
175 mg paclitaxel/1 m² = **?**/1.65 m²       **?** = 289 mg paclitaxel

*Now you try one.*

**Question:** Doxorubicin is an antineoplastic drug with many indications, including leukemia, carcinomas, and lymphomas. How many milligrams of doxorubicin would be administered in a single dose to a 20-kg, 96-cm child with leukemia if the intravenous dose is 30 mg per square meter of body surface area daily on 3 successive days every 4 weeks?

**Answer:** Utilizing the nomogram for *children*, the BSA is approximately 0.7 m². 30 mg doxorubicin/1 m² = **?**/0.7 m²       **?** = 21 mg doxorubicin

**Question:** How many milliliters of doxorubicin 2 mg/mL should be administered to provide the 4-week dosage regimen based on the *daily* dose you just calculated?

**Answer:** 2 mg doxorubicin/1 mL = 21 mg/**?**       **?** = 10.5 mL *per day*

10.5 mL/1 day = **?**/3 days       **?** = 31.5 mL every 4 weeks

# PRACTICE

1. Interpret the following medication orders/prescription Sigs:

  (a) gtt. iii o.d. q.6h, p.r.n. pain

  (b) tab i SL p.r.n. SOB

  (c) caps ii p.o. p.c. and h.s.

  (d) Humulin R® insulin 5 units SC stat

  (e) Ancef® 1 g IVPB q.6h

  (f) Inderal® 10 mg p.o., q.i.d.

  (g) Dalmane® 15 mg, cap. i, p.o., h.s.

  (h) Atrovent® inhaler, ii puffs, q.i.d., u.d.

  (i) Cortisporin Otic® gtt. ii a.u. t.i.d.

  (j) Cefzil® 250 mg/5 mL     i tsp. b.i.d. × 10 days

  (k) Persantine® 50 mg, ii tabs q.i.d., 30 min a.c.

2. Without looking back, name the seven parts of a drug order.

  (a)

  (b)

  (c)

  (d)

  (e)

  (f)

  (g)

*Questions 3–35 can all be worked by simple ratio and proportion calculations.*

3. A patient is to receive a prescription for tetracycline 250-mg capsules, and the Sig. is "cap. i p.o. q.i.d. × 10 days." How many capsules should be dispensed?

4. If the normal dose of a drug is 200 mcg, how many doses can be given from a multiple-dose vial containing 0.03 g of the drug?

5. If a patient takes diazepam 2 mg t.i.d. for 30 days, how many grams of diazepam will the patient receive after 30 days of therapy?

6. If you gave a patient a 4-fluid-ounce bottle of cough syrup and it lasted six days, how many teaspoons of the syrup did the patient take each day?

7. How many milligrams of codeine are in a tablespoonful of a medication that contains 0.36 g of codeine in a 6-fluid-ounce bottle?

8. How many milliliters of digoxin elixir containing 50 mcg/mL would provide a 0.5-mg dose?

9. A beclomethasone inhaler provides 200 inhalations, and each inhalation contains 50 mcg of the medication. How many milligrams of beclomethasone are contained in an inhaler?

10. How many milliliters of amoxicillin 125 mg/5 mL should be dispensed to a patient if the Sig. reads "1 tsp, p.o., t.i.d. × 10 days"?

**11.** How many milliliters of an injection containing 0.2 mg/mL of a drug would provide a 125-mcg dose?

**12.** If a patient purchases 2 pint bottles of an antacid and takes 2 tablespoonfuls every 6 hours, how many days will the antacid last?

**13.** An antitussive product contains 0.05 g of dextromethorphan in each teaspoonful dose. How many milligrams of dextromethorphan would be contained in a 4-ounce bottle?

**14.** How many units of heparin would a patient receive in a 24-hour period if she received 20 mL of a heparin solution containing 50 units/mL every hour?

**15.** Regular U-100 insulin contains 100 units of insulin per milliliter. If a patient administers 10 units of insulin q.i.d., how many days would a 10-mL vial last?

**16.** How many milligrams of phenytoin would a 36-lb child receive if the physician wants the child to receive 3 mg of phenytoin per kilogram of body weight?

**17.** In Question 16, how many milliliters of a phenytoin suspension containing 30 mg/5 mL should the child receive?

**18.** How many 500-mg capsules of an antibiotic are needed to provide a dosage of 25 mg/kg/day for a week for a patient weighing 220 lb?

**19.** If a 4-year-old accidentally ingested 42 5-grain acetaminophen tablets, how many milligrams of acetaminophen did the child ingest?

**20.** If the child in Question 19 weighed 44 lb, how much acetaminophen did the child ingest on a milligram-per-kilogram basis?

**21.** A patient routinely uses her metaproterenol inhaler six times a day and normally takes two puffs with each use. How many canisters of this medication should she take with her on a 42-day vacation in Europe?

> *About 200 inhalations are delivered per canister.*

**22.** If the dosage of a medication for an infant is 2 mg/lb/day, how much would a 4-kg baby receive in 5 days?

**23.** A patient received a prescription for cefaclor suspension 125 mg/5 mL. The physician failed to write a quantity to be dispensed on the prescription. According to the following directions, how many ounces should be dispensed?

Cefaclor 125/5 (Sig. 2 tsp., p.o., t.i.d. × 3d then 1 tsp., t.i.d. × 4d.)

**24.** If you were to prepare a liter of an elixir that is to contain 400 mcg of an alkaloid per tablespoonful dose, how many milligrams of the alkaloid would you need to use?

**25.** If the cost of a compounded prescription is $78.50 for a quart, how much does a $\frac{1}{2}$-fluid-ounce dose cost?

## ADVANCED PRACTICE QUESTIONS

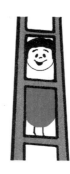

26. The dose of a drug is 0.8 mg per square meter of body surface area. How many micrograms of the drug should be administered to a child who is 42 inches tall and weighs 43 pounds?

27. The daily dose of a drug is 12 mcg per kilogram of body weight. How many milligrams of the drug would a 121-lb woman receive?

28. In the preceding question (Question 27), a prescription for 3 weeks of therapy cost the patient $285. How much does 1 milligram of the drug cost?

29. The dose of gentamicin for neonates is 2.5 mg/kg administered every 12 hours. What would be the daily dose for a 6.6-lb baby?

30. An IV solution is ordered to provide a patient 750 mL of D5W over 6 hours. How many milliliters a minute will the patient receive?

31. Digoxin injection is available in a concentration of 0.1 mg/mL. How many milliliters of injection will provide a dose of 85 mcg?

32. A patient is to receive 15 mg of Stemetil®. The drug is available as a 2-mL solution containing 25 mg of Stemetil. What volume of the solution should be administered to the patient?

**33.** The dosage of a drug is 20 mg/m²/day for 1 week. How many milligrams of the drug would a 30-year-old patient receive during the full course of therapy? (The patient is 6 feet tall and weighs 184 lb.)

**34.** An order is received for 20 mg of haloperidol decanoate to be administered by intramuscular injection. How much of a 0.05-g/mL solution should be given?

**35.** A physician orders acetaminophen 10 gr for a patient. How much of an acetaminophen 160-mg/1.6-mL solution should be given to provide the appropriate dose?

**36.** Lantus® is available in a 10 mL vial and contains 100 units/mL of insulin glargine.

   (a) How many days would a vial last a patient who receives 25 units daily at bedtime?

   (b) How many vials would a patient need to take with him on a four-month cruise around the world if he receives 30 units h.s.?

**37.** Diphenoxylate HCl and atropine sulfate tablets USP 2.5 mg/0.025 mg each contain 2.5 mg of diphenoxylate HCl and 0.025 mg of atropine sulfate.

   (a) The recommended initial dose for adults is two tablets four times daily. How many grams of atropine sulfate would an adult patient receive daily?

   (b) Teratology studies were conducted in rabbits at oral dosages of 0.4 to 20 mg/kg/day of diphenoxylate. How many micrograms of diphenoxylate would a 3.5-pound rabbit receive in the study if it received the minimum dose?

**38.** The recommended dose of infliximab is 5 mg/kg given as an intravenous induction regimen at 0, 2, and 6 weeks followed by a maintenance regimen of 5 mg/kg every 8 weeks thereafter for the treatment of adult patients with moderately to severely active ulcerative colitis.

(a) What would be the maintenance dose for a 128-pound patient?

(b) How many vials would be needed to provide the patient in part (a) with the maintenance dose if the product is available as 100 mg of lyophilized infliximab in a 20-mL vial for intravenous infusion?

**39.** Symbicort® 160/4.5 contains budesonide 160 mcg and formoterol fumarate dihydrate 4.5 mcg in each actuation.

(a) How many milligrams of budesonide are contained in a 120-inhalation canister?

(b) How many days would such a canister last if the patient received 0.009 mg of formoterol fumarate dehydrate daily?

**40.** Novolog® Mix 70/30 contains 70% insulin aspart protamine suspension and 30% insulin aspart injection and is at a concentration of 100 units/mL.

(a) How many milliliters would provide a 12-unit dose if the product is available in a 10-mL vial?

(b) If a patient receives 7 units of Novolog® Mix 70/30 a.c., what would be the percent insulin aspart protamine suspension in each injection?

*The answers to all problems can be found in the **Answer Key** beginning on page 253.*

# Reducing and Enlarging Formulas and Compounding

5

In previous chapters, I mentioned on several occasions the term **compounded prescriptions**. When I use this term, I am talking about prescriptions that are extemporaneously prepared in the pharmacy.

The term **extemporaneous** basically means spontaneous. These prescriptions are formulations that pharmacists and pharmacy technicians prepare themselves, unlike the majority of prescriptions, which are made by pharmaceutical manufacturing companies.

In years past, most prescriptions were compounded in the pharmacy, but in the latter part of the 20th century, the art of (and need for) extemporaneous compounding declined significantly. In the 1990s, however, there was a huge increase in the number of prescriptions compounded in pharmacies. This increase was due to changes in regulations and a need for more specialized and individualized pharmaceutical formulations that were not available from pharmaceutical manufacturers.

Such preparations include vaginal suppositories, dermatological ointments and creams, tablets, capsules, sterile dosage forms, and much more. In this chapter, you will learn how to interpret a prescription for compounded preparations and how to reduce and enlarge preexisting formulas to meet your needs.

*I believe the easiest way to teach the basics of compounding is by giving you different formulas as examples and following them with short discussions.*

*So let's go!*

## OBJECTIVES

Upon mastery of Chapter 5 you will be able to:

- Understand recipes for compounded prescriptions.
- Solve for the quantities required to compound a prescription.
- Enlarge a preexisting formula.
- Reduce a preexisting formula.
- Find volumes needed to compound a hyperalimentation solution.

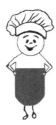

# Cooking and Compounding

**Example 1**

| Dry rice | 1 cup |
|---|---|
| Water | 2 cups |
| Salt | $\frac{1}{2}$ tsp |
| Margarine | 1 tbsp |

Combine water, salt, and margarine and bring to a boil. Add rice to boiling water, reduce heat, cover, and simmer 20 minutes.

***Makes 4 servings.***

I bet you have made something similar to this compounded product. Most of us refer to it as plain old "rice." You simply measure the different components in the formula (recipe) and mix them according to the directions to make 4 servings of rice.

**Question:**   Let's pretend you are having company over tonight and need to prepare 8 servings instead of the 4 servings this recipe makes. How much dry rice would you need to prepare the 8 servings?

**Answer:**   You probably said 2 cups of rice, because you know from experience to double the formula to get twice the amount of cooked rice. You are exactly correct with your answer, but were you aware that you were subconsciously performing a ratio and proportion calculation? Think about the solution this way:

1 cup dry rice/4 servings = $\frac{2}{8}$ servings

**Looks strangely familiar, doesn't it?**

This technique can be used for each component in the rice recipe, but there is a quicker method to enlarge a complete formula. Take the amount you need (8 servings, in this case) and divide it by the number of servings in the original formula (4). This will give you a factor of "2." Now multiply everything in the recipe by 2 to get twice as many servings.

**(For you amateur cooks: you still simmer the ingredients for only 20 minutes, not 40!)**

**Guess what?**
**You have just mastered the skill known as enlarging formulas.**

I told you this would be easy. In addition to learning how to enlarge a formula, you have already become familiar with interpreting a given recipe. By the way, did you know that there is a lot of debate about the origin of the "Rx" symbol you see on prescriptions? Many people say it stands for the word "recipe," but there are other interpretations dating back to early Greek mythology. Just thought you might want to know.

*Example 2*

**Fruit Cobbler**

| | |
|---|---|
| Biscuit baking mix | 2 cups |
| Canned fruit pie filling | 42 oz. |
| Skim milk | $\frac{3}{4}$ cup |
| Sugar | $\frac{1}{3}$ cup |
| Almond extract | $\frac{1}{4}$ tsp |

*Heat* oven to 375 degrees. *Pour* fruit into 7″ x 11″ pan. *Mix* remaining ingredients. *Drop* dough by small spoonfuls onto fruit. *Bake* 22 to 25 minutes or until golden. *Brush* with skim milk and top with sugar and cinnamon. **Makes 9 servings.**

This example is similar to Example 1 in that it is very clear what quantities are needed to prepare the fruit cobbler. However, I have another question for you.

*Question:* I'm home alone and have an incredible urge to make a small cobbler just for me. I look at the recipe and notice that it is a formula for a cobbler big enough to feed 9 people. What factor would I multiply everything by to make a "mini" cobbler big enough to feed only 3 people?

*I eat a lot!*

*Answer:* To get the conversion factor, perform the calculations in the same manner as in Example 1. Just divide the servings you need (3) by the servings in the the the formula (9).

$$\frac{3}{9} = \mathbf{0.333}$$

Your new factor is **0.333**, or $\frac{1}{3}$. Now multiply each component in the formula by $\frac{1}{3}$ to get the new formula for a "mini" cobbler.

> Don't forget that you can simply do a ratio and proportion calculation if you only need to know one component. For example, to solve for the amount of fruit in 3 servings: $\dfrac{42\,oz.}{9\ servings} = \dfrac{?}{3\ servings}$

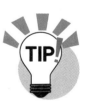

*You have mastered yet another skill, one known as reducing formulas. Now let's take a look at more pharmacy-related examples and questions.*

*Example 3*

| | |
|---|---|
| Zinc oxide | 50 g |
| Pine tar | 120 g |
| Petrolatum | 284 g |

This ointment will contain 50 g of zinc oxide, 120 g of pine tar, and 284 g of petrolatum. If you *add* all the components together, you will have a *final* preparation weighing 454 g (i.e., 1 lb). Doesn't this look just like Examples 1 and 2?

**Question:** How much pine tar would be required to prepare 1 kg of the ointment?

*Try to work this without looking at the solution.*

**Solution:** In this case, we are *enlarging* the formula to 1000 g (i.e., 1 kg) from the original formula of 454 g (i.e., 1 lb).

120 g pine tar/454 g ointment = **?**/1000 g ointment
264.3 g pine tar = **?**

> *You could also have taken the amount you need to make (1000 g) and divided it by the total grams in the original formula (454 g) to get a factor of 2.2. You can then multiply that factor by 120 to get an answer of 264 g of pine tar.*
>
> *2.2 × 120 g = 264 g pine tar*
>
> *In future problems, I will have you solve for only one component of the formula. I recommend that you utilize the ratio and proportion approach because that is how I solve the problems. In real life, you will want to solve for a factor to expedite the math process.*

**Question:** How much zinc oxide would be in 100 g of the ointment in Example 3?

**Answer:** 50 g zinc oxide/454 g ointment = **?**/100 g ointment
11 g zinc oxide = **?**

*Did you estimate your answer, or did I catch you again?*

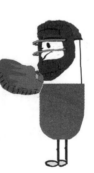

**Example 4**

| Zinc oxide | 50 |
|---|---|
| Pine tar | 120 |
| Petrolatum | q.s. ad 284 |

At first glance, this recipe looks very similar to the one in Example 3, but there are two significant differences. First, there are no units listed next to the numbers. Whenever you are compounding with *solids* and the units are not included, this usually means to use *grams*, but always double-check in case it was a careless omission. The prescriber should always include the units when ordering a compounded prescription to avoid any possible mistakes. When units are not included with *liquids,* it usually means *milliliters*, but, again, check to make sure this is what the prescriber wanted.

The second big difference is the abbreviations (q.s. and ad). The abbreviation **"q.s."** means "a sufficient quantity to make," and the abbreviation **"ad"** means "add up to."

*You will often see just one of these abbreviations, which in my opinion is plenty, but for some crazy reason people like to use both, as I have in Example 4.*

The abbreviations ad or q.s. completely alter this formula from the recipe in Example 3. In Example 3, we added all the chemicals together to get a formula weight of 454 grams. In Example 4, the final weight is 284 grams, because the ad or q.s. indicate that you will add enough petrolatum to make a final weight of 284 g.

**Question:** How much petrolatum would be required to compound the prescription in Example 4?

**Solution:** If you have 50 grams of zinc oxide and 120 grams of pine tar, then your weight is already 170 grams with just those two components. If the final weight is to be 284 grams, then simply subtract the 170 grams from 284 grams, and you will need 114 grams of petrolatum. To check your answer, add everything together and see if it all adds up to 284 grams.

> *CHECK:*    *120 g*
>              *50 g*
>       *+114 g*
>       *284 g total weight*

*To reduce or enlarge this formula, consider its total weight to be 284 grams, not 454 grams as in Example 3.*

| **Example 5** | Benzyl benzoate | 250 mL |
|---|---|---|
| | Triethanolamine | 5 mL |
| | Oleic acid | 20 mL |
| | Purified water, to make | 1000 mL |

In this recipe, the words "to make" next to the purified water mean the same thing as the abbreviation "q.s." In other words, the *final* volume of this formula will be 1000 mL. When working with liquids, you can measure all the volumes separately, but it is difficult to predict the final volume when you *add* all of them together.

For example, it is possible to add 20 mL of one chemical to 30 mL of another and wind up with a final volume of 45–55 mL. This is due to factors you need not waste brain cells learning about, but you can have volume contractions and expansions. With this in mind, you would put the 250 mL of benzyl benzoate, the 5 mL of triethanolamine, and the 20 mL of oleic acid together in a 1000-mL bottle and *add enough water to make* 1000 mL.

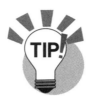

To reduce or enlarge this formula, use 1000 mL as the total volume.

**Question:**  How much benzyl benzoate would be required to prepare a pint of the lotion in Example 5?

**Answer:**  250 mL benzyl benzoate/1000 mL lotion = **?**/480 mL lotion
120 mL benzyl benzoate = **?**

Hopefully, you estimated the answer to be about half of the 250 mL.

**Question:**  How much water would you use in compounding this recipe if the words "to make" were not in the formula?

**Answer:**  You would measure 1000 mL of water and add it to the other components of the recipe. In this case, your final volume would be well above the 1000 mL you observed in Example 5.

**Example 6**

| Camphor | | |
|---|---|---|
| Menthol | a.a. | 1 g |
| Talc | | 100 g |

This is probably the most *ridiculous* abbreviation of all! The "a.a." in this prescription means "of each," which instructs you to use 1 gram of menthol and 1 gram of camphor. You will rarely see this, but I want you to recognize it in case it pops up. The reason I think this is a stupid abbreviation is because it takes no more effort to write 1 g than it takes to write a.a., so why complicate an easy process?

**Question:**  How much will the compound in Example 6 weigh?

**Answer:**  1 g camphor + 1 g menthol + 100 g talc = *102 grams*

**Example 7**

| Phenobarbital | 0.03 g |
|---|---|
| ASA | 0.6 g |
| Lactose   q.s. | |
| D.T.D. cap. #30 | |

In this prescription, the abbreviation "D.T.D." means "give of such doses." This means you are to prepare 30 capsules, with each capsule containing 600 mg of aspirin and 30 mg of phenobarbital. The q.s. next to the lactose means to add whatever quantity of lactose is necessary to fill all the capsules. *(Capsules vary in size.)*

| ***Example*** | Phenobarbital | 0.9 g |
|---|---|---|
| ***8*** | ASA | 18 g |
| | Lactose   q.s. | |
| | M. ft. cap. no. 30 | |

Here "M. ft." means to "mix and make" 30 capsules from the total weight of the two drugs, in other words, to divide the quantities in the recipe by 30 to get the amount in each capsule.

**CAUTION: Always** check whenever you have a question concerning a formula or a prescription, especially when you are unsure about the safety of a prescribed dose. With experience, you will develop clinical skills that will alert you when a dose is incorrect.

# Hyperalimentation

Frequently, pharmacy technicians will be involved in the preparation of parenteral hyperalimentation solutions, also referred to as total parenteral nutrition (TPN) solutions or just plain old "hyperal" solutions. These are complex intravenous infusions containing various nutrients, including vitamins, amino acids, dextrose, electrolytes, and trace elements. They will also frequently contain fat, insulin, and a variety of additional drugs. It is important for you to understand how to calculate hyperal solutions, even though most pharmacies today have computer programs that perform these functions.

**Partial Hyperalimentation Formula**
***(for example only)***

500 mL of 8.5% amino acid injection
0.5 L of 70% dextrose injection
Sodium chloride 35 mEq
Calcium gluconate 7 mEq
Multivitamins 5 mL
Potassium chloride 30 mEq
Sodium phosphate 9 mM
Sodium acetate 45 mEq
Ranitidine 150 mg
Vitamin K 1000 mcg
Regular insulin 8 units

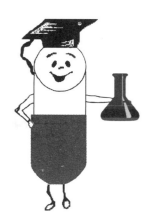

***Question:*** Determine the amount of each component source (below) required to prepare this hyperal order. Use the ratio and proportion process for each part of the question, and cover the answers to see if you can calculate them on your own.
***(Don't peek!)***

| Component source | Volume needed | Answer |
|---|---|---|
| 1-liter bottle of 8.5% amino acid injection | ___ L | 0.5 L |
| 1000-mL bottle of 70% dextrose injection | ___ mL | 500 mL |
| 30-mL vial of sodium chloride (4 mEq/mL) | ___ mL | 8.75 mL |
| 10-mL vial of calcium gluconate (4.65 mEq/vial) | ___ mL | 15 mL |
| 10-mL vial of multivitamins | ___ vials | 0.5 vial |
| 10-mL vial of potassium chloride (2 mEq/mL) | ___ vials | 1.5 vials |
| 10-mL vial of sodium phosphate (3 mM/mL) | ___ mL | 3 mL |
| 20-mL vial of sodium acetate (2 mEq/mL) | ___ 1 vial + mL | 1 vial + 2.5 mL |
| 2-mL syringe of ranitidine (25 mg/mL) | ___ syringes | 3 syringes |
| 0.5-mL amp of vitamin K (2 mg/mL) | ___ amps | 1 amp |
| 10-mL vial of regular insulin (100 units/mL) | ___ mL | 0.08 mL |

# PRACTICE

1. Without looking back, write the meaning of the following abbreviations.

   (a) a.a.                    (d) D.T.D.

   (b) ad                      (e) M.

   (c) q.s.                    (f) ft.

2. How many grams of acetaminophen would be required to prepare 5000 tablets of a narcotic analgesic if 1 tablet is to contain 10 mg of the narcotic and 325 mg of acetaminophen?

3. A cold capsule contains 30 mg of pseudoephedrine, 2 mg of brompheniramine, and 200 mg of ibuprofen. How many grams of each drug are required to make 100 of these cold capsules?

   (a) Pseudoephedrine

   (b) Brompheniramine

   (c) Ibuprofen

4. If a diphenhydramine elixir contains 12.5 mg of diphenhydramine per tea-spoon, how many grams are required to prepare a pint of the elixir?

5. An antacid tablet contains 500 mg of calcium carbonate. How many kilo-grams of calcium carbonate are required to manufacture 10,000 bottles of the antacid tablets if there are 150 tablets per bottle?

*This should keep you busy!*

6. From the following formula, calculate the number of grams of each ingredi-ent required to prepare 2 kilograms of an ointment:

   | Precipitated sulfur | 10 g |
   | Salicylic acid | 2 g |
   | Hydrophilic ointment | 88 g |

   (a) Precipitated sulfur

   (b) Salicylic acid

   (c) Hydrophilic ointment

7. From the formula in Question 6, determine how many grams of each ingredi-ent are required to prepare 60 grams of the ointment.

   (a) Precipitated sulfur

   (b) Salicylic acid

   (c) Hydrophilic ointment

**8.** How much of each ingredient is required to prepare 45 grams of the following mixture?

*These ingredients are all solids to be weighed.*

| | | |
|---|---|---|
| Camphor | | 0.3 |
| Menthol | | 2 |
| Talc | | 90 |
| Zinc oxide | q.s. | 120 |

(a) Camphor

(b) Menthol

(c) Talc

(d) Zinc oxide

**9.** From the formula in Question 8, determine how many grams of each ingredient are required to prepare 1 lb of the mixture.

(a) Camphor

(b) Menthol

(c) Talc

(d) Zinc oxide

**10.** From the following formula, determine how many milliliters of glycerin are required to prepare 1 pint of the syrup.

*These are all liquids.*

| | | |
|---|---|---|
| Glycerin | | 90 |
| Ipecac fluid extract | | 70 |
| Syrup | q.s. | 1000 |

**11.** From the formula in Question 10, determine how much ipecac fluid extract is required to prepare 1 gallon of the syrup.

**12.** The following is an old capsule formula that a veterinarian likes to use:

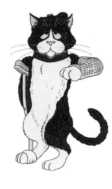

| Hydralazine | 15 mg |
|---|---|
| Reserpine | 75 mcg |
| Furosemide | 20 mg |
| D.T.D. capsules #30 | |

(a) How many milligrams of reserpine are required to prepare this prescription?

(b) How many grams of furosemide are required to fill this prescription?

(c) What is the total weight in milligrams of the three drugs in one capsule?

(d) What is the total weight in grams of the three drugs in all 30 capsules?

(e) If the prescription had *"M. ft."* instead of *"D.T.D.,"* how many micrograms of hydralazine would be in one capsule?

## ADVANCED PRACTICE QUESTIONS

**13.**

| Hydrous citric acid | | 2.1 g |
|---|---|---|
| Ferrous sulfate | | 40 g |
| Peppermint spirit | | 3 mL |
| Sucrose | | 795 g |
| Purified water | q.s. ad | 1000 mL |

(a) How many milligrams of citric acid are required to make ½ pint of this solution?

(b) How many milliliters of this solution can be made from 100 grains of ferrous sulfate?

**14.** Rx Belladonna extract      0.002
Phenobarbital                         0.03
Sodium bicarbonate            0.6
d.t.d. caps no. XXXVI

(a) How many 60-mg phenobarbital tablets are needed to prepare this prescription?

(b) How many grains of sodium bicarbonate are required to prepare these capsules?

**15.** Sucrose                        150 g
Starch                             250 g
Magnesium sulfate      0.75 g
Lactose                           125 g
Yield: 1000 placebo tablets

(a) How many kilograms of starch are needed to prepare 40,000 placebo tablets?

(b) How many placebo tablets would contain 2 lb of sucrose?

**16.** Rx Aspirin               gr V
Codeine sulfate      gr ss
d.t.d. caps #LXIV

(a) How many kilograms of aspirin are required to compound this prescription?

(b) How much would the codeine cost to prepare this prescription if 30 g cost $8.50?

**17.** Rx Acetylsalicylic acid     10 gr
    Prednisone                2.5 mg
    d.t.d. caps # XXIV

    (a) How many 5-mg prednisone tablets are required to prepare this prescription?

    (b) What is the total combined weight in grams of the drugs needed to prepare this prescription?

**18.** Do you remember my favorite question (number 35) in Chapter 1? A quick review: Tres-Lyte supplement contains $\frac{16}{100}$ g sodium, $\frac{28}{100}$ g potassium, and $\frac{25}{100}$ g phosphorus per packet and is available in boxes containing 100 3.2-g packets.

    (a) How many milligrams of inert (nonelectrolyte) filler are in each packet?

    (b) What is the ratio strength of potassium in 85 packets?

    (c) How many kilograms of phosphorus are needed to manufacture 10,000 boxes of Tri-Lyte?

    (d) How many milligrams of sodium are needed to make 30 packets?

**19.** Ipratropium bromide 0.5 mg and albuterol sulfate 3.0 mg inhalation solution is supplied as a 3-mL sterile solution for nebulization in sterile low-density polyethylene unit-dose vials and comes in cartons containing 30 vials.

    (a) How many milligrams of ipratropium bromide are required to prepare a carton of the product?

(b) How many micrograms of albuterol sulfate are contained in ½ unit dose vial?

(c) What is the percent strength of ipratropium bromide in a vial?

20. Advair® HFA 230/21 contains fluticasone propionate 230 mcg and salmeterol 21 mcg per inhalation. This inhalation aerosol is supplied in 12-gram pressurized aluminum canisters containing 120 metered actuations.

(a) How many milligrams of inert (nonmedicinal) ingredients are contained in a canister?

(b) How many kilograms of salmeterol are required to manufacture 100 canisters?

(c) This product is also available in canisters containing half the metered actuations, normally for institutional use. How many grams of fluticasone propionate are required to manufacture one of these institutional canisters?

*The answers to all problems can be found in the **Answer Key** beginning on page 253.*

**Now let's reconstitute some Dry Powders!**

# Reconstitution of Dry Powders

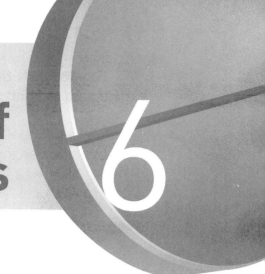

**6**

You will frequently have the opportunity to reconstitute or compound drugs that are in a dry powder form. These are usually drugs such as antibiotics that lose their potency in a short period of time after being prepared in a liquid dosage form. Because they lose their potency so quickly, it is important not to reconstitute them with water or other appropriate diluents until it is time to dispense them.

Most oral preparations are formulated so that the "normal" dose will be contained in 1 teaspoonful of the solution. In this chapter, you will learn more about compounding these dry powder products.

This morning I prepared some good old-fashioned oatmeal for breakfast. In preparing the oatmeal, I used 1 cup of dry oats and 2 cups of water. I assumed there would be about 3 cups of cooked oatmeal, but, to my surprise, there were approximately $2\frac{1}{4}$ cups. How in the world can you take 1 and add 2 and come up with approximately $2\frac{1}{4}$?

In this example, there are two things that contribute to the smaller-than-expected volume. First, some water evaporated as the mixture boiled. Second, the volume the "dry" oats displaced constricted and became much smaller when water was added. If you think about this, you will realize that dry oats have a lot of air between them, and you can compress the cup of oats to about $\frac{1}{3}$ cup simply by applying pressure. In this chapter, we will learn how to determine the volume a dry powder occupies in a reconstituted medicinal solution.

**OBJECTIVES**

Upon mastery of Chapter 6 you will be able to:

- Establish how much of a drug is contained in a vial or bottle.
- Calculate the powder volume displacement of a reconstituted drug.
- Solve problems related to dry powders.

**To establish the powder volume, simply subtract the volume of the diluent from the final volume of the solution.**

In the oatmeal example, the diluent was the 2 cups of water, and our final product was the $2\frac{1}{4}$ cups of oatmeal.

$$2\tfrac{1}{4} \text{ cups cooked oatmeal} - 2 \text{ cups water} = \tfrac{1}{4} \text{ cup}$$

This means the *powder volume* of the dry oats was actually only $\frac{1}{4}$ cup.

*You will see various formulas for solving for powder volume, but, as I stated in the Preface, I cannot stand to memorize formulas. All you need to do is use common sense and subtract from your final volume the amount of water added, and you will easily recognize the dry powder volume.*

## Reconstituting Drugs

Let's try a pharmacy-related problem.

***Question:*** Based on what you have learned in previous chapters, how much tetracycline is in a 150-mL bottle of tetracycline that says 250 mg/5 mL on the label?

***Solution:*** By now, this should be an easy problem for you.
You can solve for the answer by a simple ratio and proportion process.

250 mg tetracycline/5 mL = **?**/150 mL

7500 mg tetracycline = **?**

***Question:*** When you prepare to reconstitute (i.e., add water) to the bottle of tetracycline in the previous question, you read on the label that you must add 117 mL of water to the bottle of prepackaged tetracycline powder. Based on the information given, what is the *powder volume* of the tetracycline in the bottle?

***Solution:*** Take your final volume of 150 mL (this information is on the bottle) and simply subtract the volume of water that has been added (117 mL).

150 mL ***final volume*** – 117 mL ***water added*** = 33 mL ***powder volume***

*There are two very important points I want you to remember. These are "no-brainers" that many people fail to understand. First, the amount of the drug in the bottle never changes. In the tetracycline example, there were 7500 mg of tetracycline in the bottle. No matter whether you add 1 mL or 200 mL of water to the bottle, the amount of tetracycline remains constant; only the final volume changes. Second, the "powder volume" also remains the same. It will be 33 mL no matter what the final volume may be.*

**Question:**    In this tetracycline example, let's pretend you accidentally added 150 mL of water instead of 117 mL.

*In the "real" world of pharmacy, it would be best to throw this bottle out and start over, but please bear with me for the sake of this example and pretend you have messed up the last bottle of tetracycline in the universe!*

How much tetracycline is in the bottle?              (answer:   7500 mg)

What is the powder volume of the tetracycline?       (answer:    33 mL)

What is the final volume of the solution?            (answer:   183 mL)

**Solution:**    150 mL of water + 33 mL powder volume = 183 mL

*Now put on your thinking cap!*

How many milligrams of tetracycline are in a teaspoonful of the "messed-up" preparation?

**Solution:**    7500 mg tetracycline/183 mL = **?**/5 mL

205 mg tetracycline = **?**

How many milliliters of the "messed-up" preparation would you have to take to get the prescribed dose of 250 mg?

**Solution:**    7500 mg tetracycline/183 mL = 250 mg tetracycline/**?**

6.1 mL = **?**

*(You could also have said 205 mg tetracycline/5 mL = 250 mg/?)*

## PRACTICE

1. The label on a 200-mL bottle of ampicillin 125 mg/5 mL directs you to add 158 mL of water.

   (a) How much ampicillin is in the bottle?

   (b) What is the powder volume of the ampicillin in the bottle?

   (c) What would be the final volume if you accidentally added 178 mL of water?

   (d) How much ampicillin would be in 10 mL of the "messed-up" reconstitution in item (c)?

   (e) How many milliliters of the "messed-up" ampicillin in item (c) would be required to deliver a 250-mg dose?

2. The label on a 150-mL bottle of cefaclor 125 mg/5 mL directs you to add 111 mL of water.

   (a) How many milligrams of cefaclor are in the bottle?

   (b) What is the dry powder volume of cefaclor in the bottle?

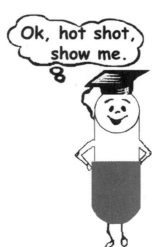

*Let's see how good you really are!*

(c) If a physician wants you to prepare a cefaclor suspension to contain 100 mg/5 mL, how much additional water would you add?

(d) Pretend you accidentally reconstituted the cefaclor bottle with 78 mL of water. How much cefaclor would be in a teaspoonful of this "incorrectly" reconstituted solution?

(e) How many milliliters of the "messed-up" cefaclor in item (d) would provide a 100-mg dose?

3. The label on a vial directs you to "add 7.8 mL of sterile water" to prepare a 10-mL "multidose" vial of a 100-mg/mL injection.

(a) How many milliliters of the reconstituted solution for injection would provide a 300-mg dose?

(b) How many grams of the drug are in one vial?

(c) If a patient is to receive 250 mg q.i.d. x 10 d. how many multidose vials will be required?

(d) What is the powder volume of the drug in this vial?

(e) How much of the reconstituted solution would provide a 250-mg dose if you accidentally reconstituted it with 9.8 mL of sterile water?

*Here is a tough one. Good luck!*

4. You are directed to reconstitute a vial of a drug. The label states that there are 10 million units of the drug in the bottle, and, when reconstituted, you will have an injection containing 500,000 units/mL.

**The drug has a dry powder volume of 7 mL.**

(a) How many milliliters of the drug will provide a 2,500,000-unit dose?

(b) How many total milliliters will be in a reconstituted bottle?

(c) How much sterile water should you add to reconstitute this injection correctly?

(d) How many units would be in 1 mL of the injection if the vial was reconstituted with 20 mL of sterile water?

(e) How much of the incorrectly reconstituted injection from item (d) would provide the 2,500,000-unit dose?

## ADVANCED PRACTICE QUESTIONS

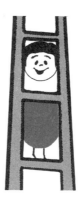

5. The label on a 15-mL bottle of azithromycin for oral suspension gives the following directions: Tap bottle to loosen powder, and add 9 mL of water.

   (a) What is the dry powder volume of the azithromycin?

   (b) How many milligrams of azithromycin are in the bottle if the label states that it contains 200 mg/5 mL?

   (c) The dosage for a 28-lb child is 100 mg daily. How many milliliters would provide a 5-day regimen for this child?

   (d) How many grams of azithromycin are in a 3.75-mL dose?

   (e) How many milliliters of the suspension would be in a bottle that was mistakenly reconstituted with 19 mL of water?

   (f) How much of the inappropriately reconstituted suspension from item (e) would provide a 100-mg dose of azithromycin?

**6.** A vial of antibiotic contains 1 gram of the drug, and the label directs you to add 3.6 mL of diluent.

(a) What is the final volume in the vial if the label says this liquid is a 250-mg/mL concentration?

(b) What is the dry volume of the drug in this vial?

(c) How many milliliters of the antibiotic would provide a 350-mg dose?

(d) How many milliliters would provide a 350-mg dose of antibiotic if the vial was reconstituted with 2.6 mL of diluent?

**7.** Amoxicillin and clavulanate potassium for oral suspension USP 400 mg/5 mL is available in a 75-mL bottle that requires 67 mL of water for reconstitution. Each teaspoonful of the liquid will contain 400 mg amoxicillin and 57 mg clavulanic acid as the potassium salt.

(a) How many grams of clavulanic acid are in a bottle?

(b) How many grams of amoxicillin would a patient receive if the patient accidentally ingested a tablespoonful dose of this medication?

(c) What volume is displaced by the dry powder?

(d) One of the recommended dosing regimens for sinusitis for patients 3 and older is 40 mg/kg/day divided every 8 hours. How many milliliters of this liquid would a 94-pound patient receive in a single dose?

(e) A technician misread the label and reconstituted this suspension with 57 mL of water instead of 67. How much clavulanic acid would be in a teaspoonful of the incorrectly prepared suspension?

(f) How many milligrams of amoxicillin would be in 3 teaspoonfuls of the incorrectly prepared suspension in item (e)?

(g) What could the technician do to correct the reconstitution mistake in item (e)?

8. Aztreonam for injection USP is supplied as single-dose, 15-mL capacity vials in two strengths: 1 g/vial and 2 g/vial. For bolus injection, the contents of a 15-mL-capacity vial should be constituted with 6 to 10 mL of sterile water.

(a) How many milligrams of aztreonam would be in the higher-strength vial if it was constituted with the highest recommended volume of sterile water for injection?

(b) What would be the ratio of aztreonam to water in the vial from item (a)?

(c) For intramuscular solutions, the contents of a 15-mL capacity vial should be constituted with at least 3 mL of an appropriate diluent per gram of aztreonam. What is the minimum volume of diluent needed to constitute the lower-strength vial for intramuscular use?

*The answers to all problems can be found in the **Answer Key** beginning on page 253.*

# Intravenous Flow Rates

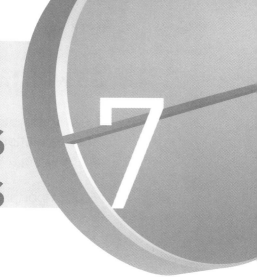

Many pharmacy technicians work in the community/retail setting and have little or no exposure to intravenous (IV) solutions. However, those of you working in hospitals and home healthcare have likely prepared numerous IV solutions. It is important for those in community practice to understand IVs because you never know when you might switch to a different area of practice in which knowledge of IVs is essential.

I know five pharmacy technicians who have made big changes in their areas of practice. The most frequent comment I hear from those technicians and from others considering a career change from retail to hospital is "I don't know anything about IVs." In fact, I know technicians who will not make a change based on that one factor. Preparing IVs is a skill you need to learn on the job or in a laboratory and is beyond the scope of this textbook.

In this chapter, I will familiarize you with math-related issues concerning IV flow rates. In later chapters, we will discuss several other topics related to intravenous solutions. Again, I will not have you learn a bunch of formulas. All the problems in this chapter will be done by simple ratio and proportion calculations.

As a pharmacy technician, you need to be aware of issues regarding flow rates, even though you will rarely determine them. Rates of delivery of IVs and other medications are usually determined by physicians in medical orders. The IVs are then administered by nurses. In many cases, pharmacists will also be involved.

## OBJECTIVES

Upon mastery of Chapter 7 you will be able to:

- Calculate the rate of delivery of IVs in milliliters per hour.
- Convert milliliter flow rates to drops per minute.
- Determine when an IV solution will run out based on flow rate.

# Go with the Flow

So why do you need to know about this flow rate stuff? Because, based on flow rate calculations, you as a pharmacy technician will have a better understanding of how long a certain IV will last before needing to be resupplied.

More importantly, by being aware of appropriate flow rates for various drugs and IV solutions, you can play an important role in assuring that mistakes are not made. I know of two critical instances in which pharmacy technicians played important roles in recognizing errors in rates of administration of drugs delivered intravenously. I also recently saw a patient die because no one caught a flow rate error.

***Now let's get to work and master flow rates.***

Large-volume parenteral solutions are usually administered to the patient either by allowing the solution to slowly drip by gravity flow into the patient's vein or through the use of electric infusion pumps. Generally, the gravitational equipment will state the **drop factor** in drops per milliliter (gtt/mL). The majority of IV administration sets deliver 10, 12, 15, 20, or 60 gtt/mL. Sets with other volumes of delivery are also available but are not as common. Electronic pumps can be set at various flow rates.

***Example:*** If an IV set is calibrated to deliver 20 gtt/mL, how many drops will deliver 60 mL of solution?

***Many people use formulas for these questions, but I bet you can work them without memorizing some crazy formula you would probably forget 3 years from now!***

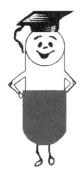

***Solution:*** Guess what? All you need to do is a ratio and proportion calculation, again!

20 gtt/1 mL = **?**/60 mL

1200 gtt = **?**

***Are you still estimating your answers?***

***Example:*** Let's look at a question from the opposite direction. What would be the "calibration" in gtt/mL of an IV infusion set that delivered 90 mL with 1350 drops?

***Solution:*** Using ratio and proportion, simply say, "If there are 1350 gtt in 90 mL, then there are **?** gtt in 1 mL."

1350 gtt/90 mL = **?**/1 mL

15 gtt = **?**

The answer 15 gtt means the IV set is calibrated to deliver 15 gtt/mL.

**Example:**   How many milliliters per minute would a patient receive if 200 mL of IV solution was being infused over a 2-hour period?

**Solution:**   I like to change the hours to minutes whenever I am asked to provide a flow rate. This is especially helpful when the question asks for *mL/min* or *gtt/min.*

> **Step 1.** 2 hours = 120 minutes
>
> **Step 2.** 200 mL/120 min = **?**/1 min
>
> > 1.67 mL = **?**

*Now let's "crank it up a notch"!*

> *Try to work this example without looking at the solution.*

**Example:**   What if an IV set calibrated at 12 gtt/mL is used? How many drops per minute would be needed to administer the IV solution in the above example?

**Solution:**   There are two ways to work this problem, and both are easy. The first solution uses the answer of 1.67 mL/min and converts it to gtt/min.

> 12 gtt/1 mL = **?**/1.67 mL
>
> 20 gtt = **?**

> This means the **1.67 milliliters per minute** is equivalent to **20 drops per minute**.

The second solution converts the original volume of 200 mL in 2 hours to drops per minute. Both solutions require two steps each, so pick your favorite one.

> **Step 1.** 12 gtt/1 mL = **?**/200 mL
>
> > 2400 gtt = **?**
>
> **Step 2.** 2400 gtt/120 min = **?**/1 min
>
> > 20 gtt = **?**

*Now it's your turn to try to put it all together. Remember that these IV drip rate problems usually require several ratio and proportion calculations, so be patient and organized.*

**Question:**   A physician writes a medication order for a liter of D5W to be administered to a patient over a 6-hour period. If the nurse uses an IV administration set that is calibrated at 10 gtt/mL, how many drops per minute should be delivered to the patient?

**Solution 1:**  Volume equals 1000 mL delivered over 360 minutes (6 hours).

> **Step 1.** 1000 mL/360 min = **?**/1 min
>
>   2.78 mL = **?**

This means that 2.78 mL will be infused each minute.

> **Step 2.** 10 gtt/1 mL = **?**/2.78 mL
>
>   27.8 gtt = **?**

This means the IV set will deliver 27.8 gtt per minute, which is the same volume as 2.78 mL. The 27.8 gtt would be rounded off to 28 gtt in the real world.

**Solution 2:**  **Step 1.** 10 gtt/1 mL = **?**/1000 mL

>   10,000 gtt = **?**

This means the liter will have 10,000 drops when using the 10-gtt/mL delivery set.

> **Step 2.** 10,000 gtt/360 min = **?**/1 min
>
>   27.8 gtt = **?**

# PRACTICE

1. A physician orders 1200 mL of normal saline to be infused in 8 hours.

   (a) How many milliliters will be infused every hour?

   (b) How many milliliters will be infused in 5 minutes?

   (c) How many drops will be in the entire volume if an IV set calibrated at 15 gtt/mL is used?

   (d) How many drops per minute must be infused using the 15-gtt/mL set to deliver the entire volume?

(e) If the solution contains 2 g of a drug, how many milligrams of the drug will the patient receive per hour?

2. A physician orders 500 mL of D5W to run for 8 hours.

   (a) Calculate the flow rate in milliliters per minute.

   (b) Calculate the flow rate in drops per minute using an infusion set calibrated at 60 gtt/mL.

   (c) If the nurse mistakenly set the flow rate at 2 mL/min, how many minutes would the solution run?

   (d) What would the drip rate be in item (c)?

   (e) If the solution contained 2 mg of a drug, how many micrograms of the drug would be in 1 mL of the solution?

3. A patient receives 40 gtt/min of an IV solution.

   (a) How many milliliters per minute does the patient receive if the nurse is using an IV set calibrated at 15 gtt/mL?

   (b) How many milliliters of fluid does the patient receive daily if the nurse is using the IV set in item (a)?

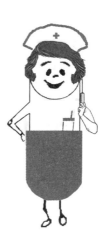

(c) Based on your answer to item (b), how many 1-liter bags of IV fluid will have to be prepared for this patient for a 24-hour period?

(d) If this solution contains 1 gram of a medication per liter, how many milligrams of the drug will the patient receive per hour?

(e) Based on the information in item (d), how many micrograms of the drug will the patient receive per minute?

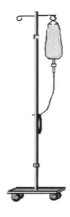

4. A physician orders a patient to receive 2 million units of ampicillin in a 1000-mL bag of an intravenous solution to be infused over 6 hours.

(a) How many milliliters of solution will the patient receive per hour?

(b) How many units of ampicillin will the patient receive per hour?

(c) How many units of ampicillin will the patient receive per minute?

(d) What is the flow rate in milliliters per minute?

(e) How many drops per hour would the patient receive if the nurse used an IV set that delivered 12 gtt/mL?

(f) How many units of ampicillin would be in a single drop of solution if an IV set delivering 12 gtt/mL was used?

**5.** A patient is to receive 100 mg of a drug per hour in an IV solution for a period of 24 hours. The total daily IV volume is 2000 mL.

(a) How many grams of the drug must the patient receive daily?

(b) How many milliliters must the patient receive per hour to get the appropriate dose?

(c) What is the flow rate in milliliters per minute?

(d) What is the flow rate in drops per minute using a venoset calibrated at 15 gtt/mL?

(e) How many milliliters of IV fluid will the patient receive in 5 hours?

(f) How many milligrams of drug will the patient receive in 3.5 hours?

## ADVANCED PRACTICE QUESTIONS

**6.** One liter of D5W ½NS is to run in an IV for 12 hours.

(a) How many milliliters will the patient receive in 3 hours and 45 minutes?

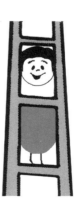

(b) How many drops per minute will the patient receive if the nurse uses an IV set calibrated at 15 gtt/mL?

**7.** An order reads: 50 mL of 10% glucose to infuse at 50 gtt/min.

   (a) How long would it take to infuse the glucose using a 60-gtt/mL infusion set?

   (b) How many liters of glucose would the patient receive every 10 minutes?

**8.** An order is written to administer 1 liter of an IV fluid over 8 hours.

   (a) How many drops per minute are required using a set calibrated at 12 gtt/mL?

   (b) How many milliliters will be infused after 1 hour?

**9.** A liter bag of normal saline was started at 10 am and is infusing at 80 mL/hr.

   (a) How long will the bag last?

   (b) At what time will the IV be completely infused?

**10.** A patient is being treated for diabetic ketoacidosis.
The label on the insulin drip states "2500 units/500 mL D5W."

   (a) How many units will the patient receive per hour if the IV infuses at 10 mL/hr?

   (b) How many drops per minute would be required to administer the units in item (a) if the IV set delivered 12 gtt/mL?

**11.** Sulfamethoxazole and trimethoprim injection USP is available in 5-mL single-dose vials containing 80 mg/mL sulfamethoxazole and 16 mg/mL trimethoprim.

(a) What is the combined weight of the drugs in a vial?

(b) Each 5-mL vial should be added to 125 mL of 5% dextrose injection. How much sulfamethoxazole would be in 50 mL of the diluted solution?

(c) The solution in item (b) should be given by intravenous infusion over 90 minutes. How many milliliters per minute should be infused?

(d) How many minutes will it take to infuse 40 mg of trimethoprim if the solution in item (b) is normally infused over 90 minutes?

(e) A physician abruptly discontinues an infusion after 38 minutes because he realizes the patient has a history of sulfa allergies. How much sulfamethoxazole has the patient already received?

**12.** Penicillin G potassium for injection is a sterile, pyrogen-free powder for reconstitution. The dose for adults with meningitis is 15 million units/day for 2 weeks. The pharmacy has this injection available only in vials containing 5,000,000 units.

(a) How many vials would be needed to provide the recommended daily dose for the full course of therapy?

(b) This antibiotic can be given by continuous intravenous drip. If a patient receives 2 L of fluid in 24 hours, how much penicillin G potassium will the patient receive in 8 hours?

(c) How many milliliters per minute will the patient receive from the intravenous drip in item (b)?

(d) How many units of penicillin G potassium will this patient receive in 100 mL of the intravenous drip in item (b)?

(e) If a set delivers 16 gtt/mL, how many drops will be required to provide 1,000,000 units of penicillin G potassium from the intravenous solution in item (b)?

*The answers to all problems can be found in the **Answer Key** beginning on page 253.*

# Percentage Calculations

**8**

An area of pharmacy math that often gives practitioners a tough time is percentage calculations. You will frequently encounter percentages in everyday pharmacy practice, so it is important to have a solid understanding of this concept. Many pharmaceutical products, from IV solutions to topicals, are labeled in percentages.

It has been my experience that pharmacy technicians and pharmacy students usually understand the concepts covered in the previous chapters but fall apart when they hit percentage calculations. My goal in Chapter 8 is to make sure you have both a firm understanding of percentages and an appreciation for them. I hope (in some perverted way) you will also have fun learning and applying the concepts in this chapter.

I know you have been exposed to the concept of percentages for many years, but do you really understand what they mean? My experience is that most people can solve basic problems related to percentages, but they are just going through the math procedures without grasping what is really going on. So if I appear to be "spoon-feeding" you in this chapter, you are very perceptive, because I am.

Now let's see what you know about basic percentages and then advance to a higher level. Oh yeah, I thought you might like to know that the math in this chapter still does not go beyond basic ratio and proportion calculations. Furthermore, there are no formulas to memorize for at least another chapter, so I am keeping my promises as much as possible.

**OBJECTIVES**

Upon mastery of Chapter 8 you will be able to:

- Define the concept of percent strength.
- Convert among percentages, fractions, decimals, and ratios.
- Solve for the quantity of a drug in a compound given its percent strength.
- Understand the different types of percentages.
- Differentiate between percent and milligram percent.
- Relate parts per million to percent strength.
- Properly write ratio strengths.

**Now let's go have fun and take the fear out of percentage calculations.**

**Example:** If you took a 100-question history final examination and got 94 questions correct, what would be your score on the exam? **Please don't tell me the answer is "an A"!**

**Solution:** I bet you correctly figured this out to be 94%, so you get your A. In this example, you simply applied the definition of **percent (%),** which is *parts per hundred,* and then solved the question. In other words, you stated:

*94 parts per 100,* **or** *94 questions per 100 questions, equals 94%*

Remember that percent means "parts per hundred," and you will easily understand the rest of Chapter 8.

Another method for solving percentage problems is to divide the number of correct answers by the *total* number of questions: $\frac{94}{100} = 0.94$.

**Wait a minute.**
How can 0.94 be 94%? If you do not understand this, then please go back to the definition of *percent*. If *percent* is defined as *parts per hundred*, the answer 0.94 means what? It means $\frac{94}{100}$, or 94 parts/100 parts. Now take the 0.94, move the decimal point two places to the right, and add a percent sign (%). This means 0.94 is exactly the same as $\frac{94}{100}$, which is exactly the same as 94%, which is exactly the same as what ratio? The answer is 94:100.

**I know, I know, it is a whole lot simpler to just say that you got an A!**

**Example:** If you are a cattle rancher in South America with 100 steers, and 65 of your steers die from cholera, what percentage of your steers die?

**Solution:** Hopefully you said 65% without a whole lot of effort. Again, we can restate these numbers in many ways. We can say 65 steers out of 100 steers **or** 0.65 **or** 65 parts out of 100 parts **or** $\frac{65}{100}$ **or** 65% **or** 65:100. These terms all mean the same thing. Oh, by the way, what ratio of steers is still alive? The answer is 35:100, which, again, is the same as $\frac{35}{100}$, 0.35, and 35%.

The percentages will always add up to 100%. In this case, 35% + 65% = 100%.

Hopefully you are still awake and understand what we have covered so far. If you have not grasped the concepts in the first two examples, do not proceed until you are very comfortable with those basic concepts of percentages. **It may be time to ask your instructor for help if this is getting confusing.** But if you are ready, then let's crank it up a notch using the same examples with a few minor changes to see if you are as smart as you think you are. I bet you are actually smarter.

***Example:*** If you took a 135-question history final examination and got 94 questions correct, what would your score on the exam be (other than bad)?

***Solution:*** You didn't do well on this exam, especially if 70% was passing. Did you calculate your score on this test to be 69.6%? If so, you are well on the way to mastering this topic, but did you think about this question as *parts per hundred,* or did you just divide 94 by 135? Right now the latter solution works, but in order to ensure that you understand later, I need you to start thinking beyond just dividing numbers. Ways to answer this question include:

$$\frac{94}{135} = 0.696 \rightarrow 69.6\%$$

### *OR*

94 questions/135 questions = **?**/100 questions

Based on years of experience, I would bet you used the first method. I prefer that you use the second, because it defines the process better. The second choice is no more difficult. It is just the plain old-fashioned ratio and proportion process. When solving this problem, did you actually think about the percentage being the number of questions you got right out of 100 instead of 135?

You probably did not, because most people rarely think of percentages on this level. Again, it will be easier for you in the long run if you solve percentages as *parts per hundred.* With this in mind, the answer 69.6% actually means that you averaged 69.6 questions right out of 100. Pretty cool, huh? Let me give you an example of how this could work in reverse.

***Example:*** If you score 69.6% on a history final examination, how many questions did you get right out of 135 questions?

***Solution:*** If 69.6% means 69.6 parts per 100, then \_\_\_\_\_ parts would be right out of 135.

$$\frac{69.6}{100} = \frac{?}{135}$$

Some people multiply 135 by 0.696 to get 94, but do they understand what is happening in this calculation? Again, I prefer the ratio method.

*Now you try one based on a previous example. Please work it by the ratio and proportion process and parts per hundred.*

**Question:**   If you are a cattle rancher in South America who had 82 steers, and 65 of your steers died from cholera, what percentage of your steers lived?

**Solution:**   If you had 82 steers and lost 65, then only 17 steers survived.

17 steers/82 *total* steers = **?**/100 steers

20.7 steers = **?**

20.7 out of 100 = ***20.7% survived***

**Question:**   In the previous question, what percentage of the steers died?

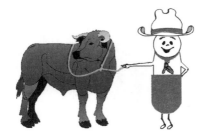

**Solution:**   100% − 20.7% = **79.3% died.**

This problem can also be solved by the ratio and proportion process:

$$\frac{65}{82} = \frac{?}{100}$$

$$79.3 = ? \quad (\frac{79.3}{100} = 79.3\%)$$

**Question:**   If another farmer lost 39% of his cattle to cholera, how many steers did he have to start with if 325 steers died?

**Solution:**   This one is a little tougher, but just think it out. What does 39% mean? It means that 39 steers died out of every 100 steers. Now set up the ratio and proportion.

39 steers died/100 steers = 325 steers died/**?**

833 total steers = **?** (i.e., the entire herd)

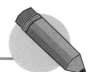

# PRACTICE

1. Find the equivalent percentage, fraction, decimal, and ratio for the following:

|  | Percent | Fraction | Decimal | Ratio |
|---|---|---|---|---|
| (a) | _____ | $\frac{3}{16}$ | _____ | _____ |
| (b) | _____ | $\frac{2}{11}$ | _____ | _____ |
| (c) | 18% | _____ | _____ | _____ |
| (d) | 3.5% | _____ | _____ | _____ |
| (e) | _____ | _____ | 0.61 | _____ |
| (f) | _____ | _____ | 0.08 | _____ |
| (g) | _____ | _____ | _____ | 1:125 |
| (h) | _____ | _____ | _____ | 35:400 |

2. Yesterday, I bought a gallon of skim milk, and I need your help:

   (a) What percentage of the milk I bought yesterday is a 12-fluid-ounce glassful?

   (b) If my wife, Patricia, drank a pint of the milk, what percentage did she drink?

*OK, so you think you are good. Try this one!*

(c) If Patricia drank a pint, my son Billy drank a quart, my daughters Kim and Angela *each* drank 6 ounces, and my baby Abby drank 120 mL, what percentage of the gallon of milk did they drink?

(d) What percentage of the milk remains for me and the dogs and cats after my family has consumed the volumes in item (c)?

**3.** Last week I took my family trout fishing, and all *six* of us caught the limit of five trout apiece. *(We fudged a little with the infant's limit!)*

(a) What percentage of the trout did each member of my family catch?

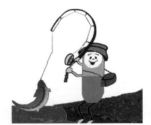

(b) What percentage of the trout did my four children catch?

(c) If the total weight of all the trout was 22.5 pounds, how many kilograms did all the trout weigh?

(d) Based on your answer to item (c), what percentage of the total weight did our largest trout weigh if it weighed 950 grams?

(e) My family had 18 trout get away after hooking them. Considering the number we caught and the number that escaped to fight another day, what percentage of the trout did we lose?

**4.** If you ate a 1-lb steak and it had a 25% fat content, how many grams of fat did you consume?

**5.** If you ate 14 ounces of pork chops and they contained 4 ounces of fat, what percentage of the pork chops was fat?

**6.** My wife, Patricia, runs marathons for fun. (I'm not really sure how running 26.2 miles can be fun, but she loves it!) She says the toughest part of the race is when she gets to the "wall," which for her is around mile number 21. What percentage of a 26.2-mile marathon has she completed when she hits the wall?

**7.** I noticed on a 448-gram can of great northern beans that the can contains 2% fat, 28 g protein, 2 g sodium, 18 g fiber, and 68 g carbohydrate.

(a) What is the percent protein in the beans?

(b) How many grams of fat are in a can of the beans?

(c) What percentage of the beans is *not* carbohydrate?

*The answers to all problems can be found in the **Answer Key** beginning on page 253.*

I bet you are wondering what all this has to do with pharmacy. Actually, we will now start relating the concepts you have (hopefully) learned to your practice setting. I want you to remember that the process of these problems doesn't change, just the context we will be working in. So goodbye to fat grams, marathons, trout fishing, and cholera-infested steers and hello to IV solutions, antifungals, glaucoma medications, and potassium supplements.

# Percentage Preparations

In pharmacy practice, you will encounter three types of percentage preparations, which are determined by the physical nature of the components in a particular product. Percentage concentrations are expressed as follows:

**Percent weight-in-weight (w/w or wt/wt)**

**Percent volume-in-volume (v/v or vol/vol)**

**Percent weight-in-volume (w/v or wt/vol)**

## Percent Weight-in-Weight (w/w or wt/wt)

This percentage expresses the number of parts of a constituent in 100 parts of a preparation. Are you wondering what a **part** is? It can be just about anything. For example, to prepare rice you could say add 1 part rice to 2 parts water. This could mean 1 cup rice to 2 cups water, or it could mean 1 handful of rice to 2 handfuls of water. Just remember, this "parts" lingo is really just talking about a ratio of one quantity to another. In the case of the rice, we want to always use twice as much water as rice, which is the same as saying "2 parts to 1 part" or "2:1."

With weight-in-weight percentages, the parts could be in grams, grains, pounds, ounces, kilograms, or any other weight measure. This type of percentage is used to measure the weight of a substance in the total weight of a product. The final product is usually a solid or a semisolid. Examples of these products are powders, ointments, and creams. This may be a little bit confusing, so let's look at a few examples.

*Example:* What would be the weight of zinc oxide (ZnO) in 120 grams of 10% zinc oxide ointment?

*Solution:* Because an *ointment* is a semisolid, it is normally **weighed,** and we usually express the weight in grams, even though other units of weight may be used. Zinc oxide is the "active" ingredient in the ointment. Zinc oxide is a solid powder, so it, too, is weighed. This problem is no different from previous examples. Just think of the grams as steers or trout, and you will do fine. I know you are going to be tempted to just multiply 10% or 0.1 times 120 g to get the answer (and that is a correct way of doing it), but I will again work the problem by that ratio and proportion process to make sure you understand the total process. Having a 10% zinc oxide ointment means that there are 10 grams of zinc oxide in 100 grams of the final ointment. So by the ratio and proportion process we can solve the problem in the following manner:

10 g **zinc oxide**/100 g **ointment** = ?/120 g **ointment**

12 g **zinc oxide** = ?

**Example:** How many grams of zinc oxide would be in 1 lb of 5% zinc oxide ointment?

**Solution:** This example is solved in the same manner as the previous one, but with one exception. When solving weight-in-weight problems, the *units must always be the same.* So you will need to convert the pound to grams.

5 g **zinc oxide**/100 g **ointment** = ?/1 lb **ointment**

5 g **zinc oxide**/100 g **ointment** = ?/454 g **ointment**

22.7 g **zinc oxide** = ?

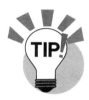

*To check your answer, take the amount of zinc oxide (22.7 g) and divide it by the total weight (454 g). 22.7/454 = 0.05 = 5/100 = 5% zinc oxide*

**Now you try to answer a couple of questions.**

**Question:** What is the percent strength of a zinc oxide ointment if you prepared 90 grams of an ointment that contains 5 grams of zinc oxide?

**Solution:** If the *final* product weighs 90 grams and contains 5 grams of zinc oxide, then to solve for the percent strength, you set up a ratio and proportion calculation to see how much zinc oxide would be in 100 g of the ointment.

5 g **zinc oxide**/90 g **ointment** = ?/100 g **ointment**

5.56 g **zinc oxide** = ?

This means there are 5.56 g of zinc oxide per 100 g of ointment, or **5.56%.**

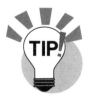

*To check your answer, just multiply 5.56% (0.0556) times 90 g to get 5 g, which is the amount of zinc oxide you used to make the ointment.*

**Now that you think you are the master of percentages, try this tricky question.**

**Question:** What would be the percent strength of a zinc oxide ointment if you *added* 90 grams of an ointment base to 5 grams of zinc oxide?

**OOPS! Didn't I just ask you this question?**

***Solution:*** Contrary to what you might think, this is **not similar** to the previous question.

In the other question, I said that the 90 g of ointment *contained* the 5 g of zinc oxide. In this question, I said that you *added* 5 grams of zinc oxide *to* **90** grams of an ointment base.

In the first question, the final weight was 90 grams, but in this one, the final weight is **95** grams.

5 g **zinc oxide**/95 g **ointment** = **?**/100 g **ointment**

5.26 g **zinc oxide** = **?**

5.26/100 = 5.26%

# PRACTICE

8. If you were to prepare 150 g of a coal tar ointment containing 12 g of coal tar,

   (a) What would be the percent strength of coal tar in the ointment?

   (b) What would be the percent strength of coal tar in 1 mg of ointment?

9. If you prepare a powder that contains 2 mg of a drug in every gram of powder,

   (a) How much of the drug will be in 120 grams of the powder?

   (b) What is the percent strength of the drug in the powder?

**10.** If you were to prepare a topical cream containing 3% hydrocortisone,

   (a) How many grams of hydrocortisone would be required to prepare 1 pound of the topical cream?

   (b) How many milligrams of hydrocortisone would be in 1 g of the cream?

**11.** If 25 grams of Efudex® Cream contains 5% fluorouracil,

   (a) How many milligrams of fluorouracil are in the cream?

   (b) What would be the new percent strength if you *added* 2 g of fluorouracil to the Efudex Cream?

**12.** From the following formula:

| | |
|---|---|
| Hydrocortisone | 1.5 g |
| Vioform powder | 0.5 g |
| Cream base        ad | 60 g |

   (a) What is the percent strength of hydrocortisone in this cream?

   (b) How much cream base is required to prepare this prescription?

   (c) How much Vioform® powder is required to prepare 10 ounces of this cream?

**13.** From the following formula:

| | |
|---|---|
| Phenobarbital Na | 60 mg |
| Aminophylline | 200 mg |
| Carbowax base | 1.8 g |

(a) This formula is for one suppository; how many grams of aminophylline are required to prepare 60 suppositories?

(b) How much would the 60 suppositories weigh?

(c) What would be the percent strength of phenobarbital in 60 suppositories?

**14.** From the following formula:

| | |
|---|---|
| Benzocaine | 1:1000 |
| Precipitated sulfur | 10% |
| Zinc oxide paste | ad 120 g |

(a) How many milligrams of benzocaine are in this prescription?

(b) How many grams of precipitated sulfur would be required to prepare a kilogram of this product?

**15.** From the following formula:

| | |
|---|---|
| Magnesium oxide | 2 parts |
| Sodium bicarbonate | 5 parts |
| Calcium carbonate | 7 parts |

(a) How many grams of calcium carbonate are required to prepare 2 pounds of this powder?

(b) What is the percent strength of sodium bicarbonate in the powder?

(c) What is the ratio strength of magnesium oxide in the powder?

*The answers to all problems can be found in the **Answer Key** beginning on page 253.*

# Percent Volume-in-Volume (v/v or vol/vol)

A second type of percentage is percent volume-in-volume. You will not see this type of percentage very often, but you still need to have a working knowledge of such problems. Fortunately, percent v/v problems are worked in a similar manner as percent w/w problems. In the previous section, we discussed weight-in-weight percentages in which the active constituent (the drug) was weighed and the final product was a solid and was also weighed.

The percent volume-in-volume compounds are solution or liquid preparations, and the active constituents are also solutions or liquids. In most cases, we will measure the volumes of the final products and the constituents in milliliters. These types of problems also can be worked with other units of volume (i.e., pints, fluid ounces, or quarts), but please do not forget that all units must be the same, just as we saw in the weight-in-weight problems.

**Example:** What is the percent strength (v/v) of a pint of a solution that contains 1 fluid ounce of liquefied phenol?

**Solution:** Just as you did with the percent w/w problems, simply put everything into the same units and solve for parts per 100 to get the percentage. In this example, a pint equals 480 mL, and a fluid ounce contains 30 mL.

30 mL **liquefied phenol**/480 mL **solution** = ?/100 mL **solution**

6.25 mL **liquefied phenol** = ?

*Every 100 mL of the solution contains 6.25 mL of liquefied phenol. 6.25 mL/100 mL = 6.25% (v/v)*

*You also could have said 30/480 = 0.0625 = 6.25%, but I still want you to work these problems by the ratio and proportion process.*

*Do you see an easier way to work this example? You could have said that a pint has 16 fluid ounces, and the solution contains 1 fluid ounce of liquefied phenol.*

*1 fl.ounce/16 fl.ounces = ?/100 fl.ounces*

*6.25 fl.ounces = ?*

# PRACTICE

**16.** A mouthwash contains 0.35% (v/v) of a mint flavoring.

    (a)  How many milliliters of flavoring are in a quart of the mouthwash?

    (b)  If you have a gallon of this mouthwash, what would be the percent strength (v/v) of mint flavoring in 1 mL of the mouthwash?

**17.** Six fluid ounces of a lotion contain 16 mL of resorcinol monoacetate.

    (a)  What is the percent strength of resorcinol monoacetate in this lotion?

    (b)  How many milliliters of resorcinol monoacetate are required to prepare 5 liters of the lotion?

**18.** You have 1 pint of methyl salicylate available.

    (a)  How many gallons of a 6% methyl salicylate lotion can you prepare?

    (b)  How many milliliters of methyl salicylate are needed to prepare a pint of 6% methyl salicylate lotion?

**19.** If verigreen spirits contain 5% verigreen oil, how many milliliters of the spirits can be prepared from a tablespoonful of verigreen oil?

**20.** If dynamint spirits contain 1:15 dynamint oil, how many milliliters of the spirits can be prepared from $\frac{1}{2}$ pint of dynamint oil?

*The answers to all problems can be found in the **Answer Key** beginning on page 253.*

# Percent Weight-in-Volume (w/v or wt/vol)

Last, but not least, is percent weight-in-volume, a percentage you will frequently work with in most practice settings. As with the volume-in-volume percentage problems, the final product in w/v problems is a solution or liquid preparation. The big difference is that the constituent or drug is measured by weight.

By now you have probably noticed a trend. In the abbreviations (w/w, v/v, and w/v), the denominator tells you if the final product is a solid or a liquid (i.e., whether it is measured by weight or by volume), and the numerator gives you the same information about the constituent or drug. Unfortunately, you will rarely see these abbreviations next to a percent sign in the real world of medicine and pharmacy.

You will eventually learn from experience how to recognize the different types of percentages. In percent volume-in-volume (v/v) solutions, you may recall, the units could vary as long as they were the same kind of units. You could have pints per pints, milliliters per milliliters, or quarts per quarts. In the percent weight-in-weight (w/w) preparations, the units could also vary but had to be the same kind of units. You could have g/g, kg/kg, lb/lb, gr/gr, and so on. This is **not** the case with percent weight-in-volume. With percent w/v, the numerator or constituent is measured in grams only, and the denominator or final solution is measured in milliliters only. An example of this would be a solution of 10% potassium chloride (KCl). The 10% here means 10 grams KCl/100 milliliters solution.

**Example:** What would be the percent w/v of a solution of potassium chloride that contained 24 grams of potassium chloride in 4 fluid ounces?

**Solution:** Do not forget to **always** solve these problems with *grams* of constituent over *100 milliliters* of final solution. In this example, we have 24 g/4 fl. oz. This needs to be changed to 24 **g**/120 **mL**.

24 **g KCl**/120 **mL solution** = ?/100 **mL solution**

20 **g KCl** = ?

20 g/100 mL = 20% (w/v)

**Example:** How many grams of potassium chloride would be in a pint of 10% KCl?

**Solution:** Change the pint to 480 mL. Ten percent means 10 g KCl/100 mL.

10 **g KCl**/100 **mL solution** = ?/480 **mL solution**

48 **g KCl** = ?

In other words, if there are 10 g of KCl in 100 mL of the 10% solution, then there must be 48 g of KCl in 480 mL of the solution.

## PRACTICE

**21.** You have a liter bag of normal saline (NS) that is 0.9% sodium chloride.

(a) How many grams of sodium chloride are contained in the bag?

(b) If a patient receives 200 mL of the NS every hour, how many milligrams of sodium chloride will he receive in 3 hours?

**22.** A ½ liter IV solution contains 37.5 grams of sodium bicarbonate.

(a) What is the percent strength of sodium bicarbonate in the solution?

(b) How many milligrams of sodium bicarbonate are in 100 mL of the solution?

(c) What is the percent sodium bicarbonate in 5 mL of the IV solution?

**23.** You have on hand 85 grams of iodine.

(a) What would be the percent strength of a gallon of iodine tincture compounded with the 85 grams?

(b) How many milliliters of 3% iodine tincture can be made from the amount of iodine on hand?

(c) How much of a 1:100 iodine tincture can be made from the amount of iodine on hand?

*The 1:100 ratio means 1 g:100 mL.*

**24.** Adenosine phosphate is available in 10-mL vials that contain 25 mg/mL.

(a) How many grams of adenosine phosphate are in a vial?

(b) What is the percent strength of adenosine phosphate?

(c) How many milliliters of adenosine phosphate would provide a 0.035-g dose?

**25.** Pilocarpine is available as a 0.5% solution.

(a) How many milligrams of pilocarpine are required to prepare 15 mL of the pilocarpine solution?

(b) If the dropper bottle delivers 18 drops of 5% pilocarpine solution in each milliliter, how many drops are in a 15-mL bottle of pilocarpine?

(c) Based on your answers to items (a) and (b), how many micrograms of pilocarpine are contained in 1 drop of the solution?

**26.** If 50 milligrams of nitroglycerin are in a liter of IV fluid:

(a) What is the percent strength of nitroglycerin?

(b) How many milliliters of the solution would deliver a 200-mcg dose?

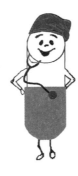

**27.** If a physician ordered a 15-mg "test dose" of a drug for a patient, how many milliliters of a 5% solution would be used to provide the dose?

*The answers to all problems can be found in the **Answer Key** beginning on page 253.*

## Milligram Percents (mg%)

If you are working in an institutional environment, you will sometimes see another type of percentage referred to as a milligram percent (mg%). These milligram percents are not routinely used for dosing, but they are frequently used in reporting various clinical laboratory test results. They are used to report various chemicals that are present in the body in small quantities, such as cholesterol, glucose, creatinine, and even some drugs.

In the last section, you learned about weight-in-volume percentages, which were measured as g/100 mL. The only difference with milligram percent problems is that the numerators are in milligrams instead of grams. Also, instead of seeing 100 mL in the denominator, you will see the letters dL. These letters stand for a "deciliter," which is the same as 1/10 of a liter, which is the same as 100 mL.

*So we are back to where we started!*

**Example:**    If a patient's serum glucose is reported as 165 mg/dL, express this value as a mg%.

**Solution:**    Remember that a deciliter (dL) equals 100 mL.

165 mg/dL = 165 mg/100 mL = *165 mg%*

**Example:**    Express 165 mg% as a normal weight-in-volume percentage.

**Solution:**    If 165 mg equals 0.165 g, then you could say the following:

165 mg% = 165 mg/100 mL = 0.165 g/100 mL = *0.165%*

# PRACTICE

**28.** In most states, you would be considered legally drunk if you had a blood alcohol level of 200 mg/dL. Express this as a normal percentage (w/v).

**29.** A patient has a serum creatinine of 0.15% (w/v). Express this as a mg%.

**30.** If a patient has a serum cholesterol level of 95 mg%, how many micrograms of cholesterol will be in 1 mL of serum?

*The answers to all problems can be found in the **Answer Key** beginning on page 253.*

## Parts Per Million (ppm)

As you saw in the last section, mg% is used to measure very small quantities. It is easier and safer to write 5 mg% than 0.005%. In this section, we will see a term that is used for even more dilute solutions than mg%. The term is parts per million (ppm). Probably the most common example of a substance measured in ppm is the fluoride in your drinking water. If your drinking water contains 2 ppm, this indicates that there are 2 grams of fluoride in every "million" milliliters of water. This concentration can also be written as a ratio: 2:1,000,000. As you can see, 2 ppm is less difficult to write than 0.0002%. The term ppm can also be used for weight-in-weight and volume-in-volume problems.

## PRACTICE

**31.** An antifungal is available in dry fish feed in a concentration of 8 ppm.

    (a) Express this concentration as a ratio (reduce to lowest terms).

    (b) Express this concentration as a percentage (w/w).

    (c) How many grams of antifungal would be in a kilogram of the feed?

**32.** How many grams of sodium fluoride would be required to prepare 1000 gallons of a 1-ppm supply of fluoridated drinking water?

**33.** Express 0.00005% (w/v) in parts per million.

**34.** How many micrograms would be in a liter of the solution in question 33?

*The answers to all problems can be found in the **Answer Key** beginning on page 253.*

## Writing Ratio Strengths

Until now I have been letting you get away with writing ratios any way you wanted to because I wanted you to understand the basic concepts behind percentages, fractions, and ratios. Now it is time for you to learn the proper format for writing ratios. This is a very simple process that, once again, uses the ratio and proportion process.

To write ratios properly, you should always have a 1 to the left of the colon. In other words, 5:25 would be incorrect. The correct way of writing this ratio would be 1:5. In this example, we just divided both sides by 5 and reduced to lowest terms. But what would you do if the ratio was 5:13? To set this problem up correctly, plug your numbers into another ratio and proportion calculation using a 1 above the **?**. By doing this, the **1** will represent the number to the left of the colon, and the number you get for the **?** will represent the number to the right of the colon. This is how it will look:

$$\frac{5}{13} = \frac{1}{?} \qquad \text{(or } 5:13 \text{ equals } \mathbf{1:?})$$
$$2.6 = ?$$

The ratio $\frac{5}{13}$ or 5:13 now becomes 1:2.6.

To check your answer, divide both fractions, and you will get the same decimal answer: 5 divided by 13 equals 0.3846, and 1 divided by 2.6 equals 0.3846.

# PRACTICE

**35.** Convert the following numbers to correctly written ratios:

(a) 2/7

(f) 0.45

(b) 17/510

(g) 2:23

(c) 33/135

(h) 23:300

(d) 0.125

(i) 48:200

(e) 0.08

## ADVANCED PRACTICE QUESTIONS

**36.** The concentration of a pesticide in animal feed is 6 ppm.

(a) How many kilograms of animal feed contain 1 mg of pesticide?

(b) Express the concentration of pesticide in animal feed as a ratio strength.

**37.** Rx    Potassium permanganate solution    3 liters
                                              1:1000

(a) How many tablets containing 0.5 g of potassium permanganate are required to prepare this prescription?

(b) What will be the percent strength of the solution if you incorrectly use 60 of the 0.5-g tablets?

**38.** Rx    Resorcinol lotion    10%
Sig.    Apply as directed

(a) How many milliliters of resorcinol monoacetate should be used in preparing $\frac{1}{2}$ L of lotion?

(b) What is the ratio strength of 8.35 mL of the lotion?

**39.** Pediatric atropine sulfate has a concentration of 0.05 mg/mL.

(a) Express this concentration as a mg%.

(b) How many micrograms of atropine sulfate will be in a 5-mL syringe?

**40.** Bupivacaine hydrochloride 0.5% and epinephrine 1:200,000 injection is available as a 30-mL single-dose vial and is used for nerve block and for caudal and epidural anesthesia.

(a) How many milligrams of bupivacaine are contained in a vial of the solution?

(b) How many micrograms of epinephrine are contained in 1 mL of the solution?

**41.** *Do you remember this next one from Chapters 1, 2, 3, and 5?*

Tres-Lyte supplement contains 160 mg sodium, 280 mg potassium, and 250 mg phosphorus per packet. Tres-Lyte is available in boxes of 100 packets, each weighing 3.2 g.

(a) What is the ratio strength of sodium in a packet?

(b) What is the percent strength of phosphorus in a packet?

**42.** Timolol maleate ophthalmic solution is available in a 0.25% strength.

(a) How many milligrams of timolol maleate are in 5 mL of this solution?

(b) What is the ratio strength of timolol maleate in 5 mL?

**43.** Midazolam injection USP is available in various strengths, including a flip-top vial containing 5 mg midazolam in 1 mL of injection.

(a) What is the percent strength of midazolam in the vial?

(b) How many grams of midazolam are required to manufacture 20 L of this injection?

**44.** Lidocaine hydrochloride topical solution USP 4% contains a local anesthetic agent and is administered topically. It is supplied in 50-mL and 100-mL bottles.

(a) What would be the ratio strength of combining both size bottles?

(b) How many milligrams of lidocaine hydrochloride would be delivered if 3 mL of the solution was applied?

**45.** Dexamethasone tablets USP are available in strengths of 0.5, 0.75, 1, 1.5, 2, 4, and 6 mg.

(a) What would be the resulting milligram percent of a solution made by dissolving one tablet of each strength in 30 mL of a solvent?

(b) What is the ratio strength of the solution in item (a) above?

*The answers to all problems can be found in the **Answer Key** beginning on page 253.*

# Concentrations and Dilutions

**9**

Please *do* not *continue until you have mastered Chapters 1 through 8. This chapter is based on your having a strong understanding of previous information, especially information related to ratios and percentages.*

There will be times when you will have to **compound** by reducing the strength of a **concentrated** (stock) product to a lower strength. This procedure is known as a **dilution.** Examples of dilution are preparing a 5% IV solution from a 10% solution or preparing a 2% ointment by mixing 1% and 3% ointments.

In Chapter 9, I will teach you how to handle dilutions with as little pain as possible. Because of the uniqueness of dilutions, I have to veer a little from the ratio and proportion technique. In addition, I have to use a formula. I hate to do this, but hopefully you will forgive me once you become a dilution master!

I would confidently bet that you have solved for the **average** of something during your tenure on earth! One thing that comes to mind are your grades in school. Now, I am going to assume you are pretty bright, because you are already in Chapter 9 of this book.

As an example, why don't we figure out your average in an English course?

## OBJECTIVES

Upon mastery of Chapter 9 you will be able to:

- Solve for the average percent strength of a mixture using alligation medial.
- Determine the amount of a stock solution required to prepare a dilution.
- Perform dilutions of liquid, semisolid, and solid dosage forms.
- Explain how to determine mixture proportions using alligation alternate.
- Calculate volumes and weights using specific gravity.

**Example:** What would your English average have been if you had scored 80%, 90%, and 100% on three tests?

**Solution:** Hopefully, you added the numbers and divided by 3.

    **Step 1.** 80 + 90 + 100 = 270

    **Step 2.** 270 ÷ 3 = **90%** (your average score)

*Now you try solving several problems for the average.*

**Question:** What would be the average weight of a steak if you bought four steaks that weighed $\frac{3}{4}$ pound, $\frac{1}{2}$ pound, $2\frac{1}{2}$ pounds, and 20 ounces?

**Solution 1** There are two ways to solve this question, and both require that all units be equal. In Solution 1, let's convert everything to pounds:

$\frac{3}{4}$ lb + $\frac{1}{2}$ lb + $2\frac{1}{2}$ lb + $1\frac{1}{4}$ lb = 5 lb

*Convert 20 ounces to pounds by saying: 16 oz/1 lb = 20 oz/?*
*$1\frac{1}{4}$ lb = ?*

5 lb ÷ 4 steaks = an average of $1\frac{1}{4}$ lb per steak

*In a ratio and proportion calculation, you would say, "If 4 steaks weigh 5 pounds, then 1 steak would weigh (?) pounds.*
*4 steaks/5 lb = 1 steak/?*
*$1\frac{1}{4}$ lb = ?*

**Solution 2** For this second solution, I again convert the weight of each steak to the same units. This time, I convert the pounds to ounces. Again, all I need to do is a simple ratio and proportion calculation.

**Example:** 1 lb/16 oz = $\frac{3}{4}$ lb/**?**

12 oz = **?**

Now add all the ounces and divide by 4 steaks.

12 oz + 8 oz + 40 oz + 20 oz = 80 oz

80 oz ÷ 4 steaks = *20 oz per steak (the same as $1\frac{1}{4}$ lb per steak)*

**Question:** My family has three cars (one doesn't run) that have varying fuel capacities. My wife's car holds 23.5 gallons of gasoline, my car holds 62 quarts, and the car that doesn't run holds 96 pints. What is the cars' average fuel capacity?

**Solution:** Again, you need to convert to one unit. For this example, let's convert to quarts. Our answer will be the same if we convert to pints or to gallons.

4 qt/1 gal = **?**/23.5 gal      **? = 94 qt**

 2 pt/1 qt = 96 pt/**?**      **? = 48 qt**

Now add the quantities and divide by 3.

62 + 94 + 48 = 204 quarts (the total for all three cars)

204 ÷ 3 = 68 quarts (*the average fuel capacity*)

## Alligation Medial

*Instead of an explanation, let's look at an example.*

**Example:** Assume you move into a new seven-room home and decide to put telephones in every room except the two bathrooms. What would be the average cost of a telephone if you paid $32 for the family-room phone, $48 for the kitchen phone, and $22 each for the three bedroom phones?

**Solution:** The hard way to work this problem is: $32 + $48 + $22 + $22 + $22 = $146

$146 ÷ 5 = *$29.20 per phone*

*There is an easier way. Did you think of it?*

| | | | | |
|---|---|---|---|---|
| 1 phone | × | $32 | = | $32 |
| 1 phone | × | $48 | = | $48 |
| + 3 phones | × | $22 | = | $66 |
| **5 phones** | | | | **$146** |

**5 phones/$146 = 1 phone/?** or $146/5 phones = $29.20
= cost of 1 phone

*Guess what? This second solution is alligation medial, so you already know this technique!*

*Now let's apply it to the world of pharmacy practice.*

# PRACTICE

1. What is the average number of prescriptions that can be filled daily by the pharmacy technicians at a large city hospital if 12 technicians can each fill 100 prescriptions each day, 20 can each fill 125 prescriptions, 23 can each fill 150 prescriptions, and 8 can each fill 175 prescriptions?

2. What is the percent alcohol in a mixture of 2 liters of 20% alcohol, 1 liter of 50% alcohol, and 750 mL of 80% alcohol?

3. What is the percent concentration of potassium chloride in a mixture of 1 pint of 10% KCl, 3 quarts of 5% KCl, and 1 gallon of 20% KCl?

4. What would be the final percent strength of potassium chloride if you added 1 quart of water to the mixture in question 3?

5. What is the percent strength of benzalkonium chloride in a mixture of 1 pint of 2% benzalkonium chloride and 1 liter of 6% benzalkonium chloride?

6. What would be the final percent concentration of benzalkonium chloride if you added $\frac{1}{2}$ liter of a 1:500 benzalkonium chloride solution to the mixture in Question 5?

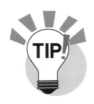

*I highly recommend converting ratios to percentages before working any of these dilution problems.*

**Now I bet I can trick you!**

7. What is the percent strength of alcohol in a mixture of a liter of 95% alcohol, a quart of 70% alcohol, and a pint of 17% benzalkonium chloride?

*Benzalkonium chloride is 0% alcohol.*

8. What is the percent strength of ichthammol in a mixture of 100 grams *each* of ichthammol ointments containing 5%, 15%, and 20%?

9. What would be the ratio strength of ichthammol in the ointment in question 8 if you added 100 grams of pure ichthammol?

   *(For the purposes of this question, consider "pure" ichthammol to be 100%.)*

10. What would be the percent strength of a mixture of 1 lb of a 1:50 sulfur powder and 1 kg of a 1:20 sulfur powder?

*The answers to all problems can be found in the **Answer Key** beginning on page 253.*

*Are you still estimating your answers?*

*If not, shame on you!*

## Stock Solutions and Dilutions

Stock solutions are "concentrated" or "potent" solutions of medicinal substances that are frequently used to compound "weaker" solutions for human use. These stock solutions are very convenient, because a pharmacist or pharmacy technician can prepare very large volumes of a product from small volumes of the stock solution.

You have probably used a form of a stock solution on several occasions in your home. Examples at my home are insecticides, hardwood floor cleaners, hummingbird food, weed killer, and plant fertilizer. All of these products are in small bottles of concentrate that require dilution with water. Such products would be dangerous to use without diluting. The advantage of stock solutions is that they save you tons of space. In this section, we will learn how to prepare dilutions using stock solutions and other concentrates.

**PLEASE NOTE:** *Dilutions cannot be worked by simple ratio and proportion calculations, because there is an inverse relationship occurring, so your answer will be way off base! Always, always, always estimate your answers, especially when you are working dilution problems.*

*Now let's have some fun diluting!*

The formula I like best for solving dilutions is:    **(OV) (O%) = (NV) (N%)**

I know this looks complicated, but it is a very easy formula to remember. The abbreviations stand for the following:

**OV** stands for **O**ld **V**olume *(This is the volume we are starting with.)*

**O%** stands for **O**ld *% (This is the percent concentration of the **O**ld **V**olume.)*

**NV** stands for **N**ew **V**olume *(This is the "new" volume you are making.)*

**N%** stands for **N**ew *% (This is the "new" percent of the **NV** after the dilution.)*

Let's take a look at several examples to better explain what all this stuff means. You will know you are doing a dilution when you are taking a solution with a high percent strength and adding a diluent like water to "dilute" it down to a lower percent strength, or "weaker," solution. It is very important to pay attention to the wording of this kind of question so that you can spot dilution problems when they appear. Otherwise, you might try to work these problems incorrectly with the ratio and proportion method.

**Example:**    How many milliliters of a 20% *stock* solution of drug T would you need to prepare 500 mL of a 3% solution of drug T?

**Solution:**    When reading a problem like this, you should first note that you are taking a concentrated solution (20%) and compounding a weaker solution (3%). By definition, you know this is a *dilution* and you had better **not** use the ratio and proportion process to solve it. You also should estimate your answer. In this example, I know that if I am making 500 mL of a weaker solution, I will be using some quantity of the 20% concentrate less than 500 mL to prepare it. Now let me show you what a gazillion of my pharmacy students try to do.

**Please note that this is the incorrect way to work this problem!**

3%/500 mL = 20%/**?**

3333 mL = **?**

*Not even close to the correct answer !!!!*

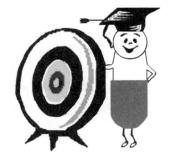

*Now let's work it CORRECTLY.*

$$(OV)(O\%) = (NV)(N\%)$$

We want to solve for **(OV)**, or the volume of the **stock solution**. Just as with ratio and proportion calculations, if you know three things, you can easily solve for the fourth, which in this case is **(OV)**. In this problem, and in all dilution problems, you will know three factors. In this problem, you know that **(O%)** is 20%, **(NV)** is 500 mL, and **(N%)** is 3%.

Now, just plug everything into the "magical" formula and solve for the missing number:

$$(OV)(O\%) = (NV)(N\%)$$

$$(OV)(20\%) = (500 \text{ mL})(3\%)$$

$$(OV) = (500 \text{ mL})(3\%)/(20\%)$$

$$(OV) = 1500 \text{ mL}\%/20\%$$

$$(OV) = 75 \text{ mL}$$

The 75-mL answer means you would measure 75 mL of the 20% stock solution and *add* enough water to it *to make* 500 mL of a 3% solution.

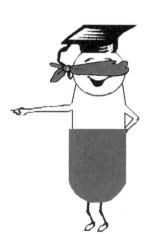

Now I have three questions to see if you really understand the example we just solved. *Cover the correct solutions*, and try to answer these questions as well as you possibly can.

**Question 1**  Approximately how much water will you add to the 20% solution of drug T to make this dilution?

**Answer:**  Approximately 425 mL of water must be *added*. If the final volume is 500 mL and you are going to use 75 mL of the 20% stock solution, then 500 minus 75 equals 425 mL. The reason I say *approximate* is because you are going to take the 75 mL of 20% solution and q.s. (add enough water) to make 500 mL. The true volume may be a little more or a little less than 425 mL, but this is close enough!

**Question 2**  Which volume has more of drug T in it, 75 mL of the 20% solution or 500 mL of the 3% solution?

**Answer:**  Both volumes will have *exactly* the same amount of the drug in them. Do not forget, the 500-mL solution was prepared from the 75 mL of stock solution, so whatever amount of the drug was in the 75 mL is also in the 500 mL. If you still do not believe me, check your answers as a percentage using the ratio and proportion process.

*For the 75 mL of 20% solution:*     20 g **drug T**/100 mL = **?/75 mL**

                                      15 g **drug T** = **?**

*For the 500 mL of 3% solution:*     3 g **drug T**/100 mL = **?/500 mL**

                                      15 g **drug T** = **?**

**Question
3**

Since the 75-mL and 500-mL solutions each contain 15 g of drug T, there will also be the same amount of drug T in a teaspoon of each solution.

**TRUE or FALSE?**

**Answer:**

The answer is a really big **false**. Even though both solutions, the 75 mL and the 500 mL, contain the same amount of drug, their *concentrations* of drug T are very different. One solution contains 15 g of the drug in 75 mL, and the other has 15 g in 500 mL.

The **concentrated** solution will contain:
  15 g **drug T**/75 mL = **?/5 mL**
          1 g **drug T** = **?**

This means there will be 1 g of drug T in each teaspoon of the *concentrate*.

The **diluted** solution will contain:
  15 g **drug T**/500 mL = **?/5 mL**
         0.15 g **drug T** = **?**

This means there will be 0.15 g of drug T in each teaspoon of the *dilution*.

*Now let's try a few more questions using our formula but solving for other missing factors. Again, please try to work these problems before looking at the solutions.*

**Question:**

What is the percent sucrose in a solution if 100 mL of 50% sucrose is diluted to a pint with water?

**Solution:**

**(OV) (O%) = (NV) (N%)**

(100 mL) (50%) = (480 mL) (N%)

5000 mL%/480 mL = (N%)

**10.42% = N%**

**Question:**

What is the percent sucrose in a solution if 100 mL of 50% sucrose is added to a pint of water?

*Did I just ask you this same question?*

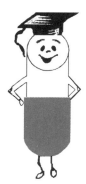

*(If you said yes, then I suckered you into a common error many people make. In the first question, the final volume is 480 mL, but in this question, the final volume is 580 mL, because I said you added 100 mL to 480 mL. If I did not trick you here, then you are far brighter than my average student!)*

*The message is: READ CAREFULLY.*

**Solution:**  **(OV) (O%) = (NV) (N%)**

(100 mL) (50%) = (580 mL) (N%)

5000 mL%/580 mL = (N%)

**8.62% = N%**

# PRACTICE

**11.** A fluid ounce of 10% boric acid is diluted to a liter with water.

(a) What is the percent strength of the dilution?

(b) What is the ratio strength of the dilution?

(c) How much boric acid is in a tablespoonful of the dilution?

(d) How much boric acid was in a teaspoonful of the concentrated solution before the dilution was made?

**12.** You have 4 fluid ounces of 10% aluminum acetate solution available in your pharmacy as a stock solution.

   (a) How many milliliters of a 1:100 solution of aluminum acetate can be prepared from the volume you have on hand?

   (b) Approximately how much water would you *add* to the stock solution to prepare the dilution in item (a)?

**13.** How many milliliters of a 17% benzalkonium chloride stock solution are needed to prepare a liter of a 1:200 solution of benzalkonium chloride?

**14.** How many milligrams of benzalkonium chloride are in a fluid ounce of the dilution prepared in Question 13?

**15.** What is the percent strength of a stock solution if you took 10 mL of the stock solution, diluted it to a liter with water, and had a final dilution strength of 0.5%?

**16.** How many grams of the chemical would be in a pint bottle of the stock solution in Question 15?

**17.** You have a 4-ounce tube of a 5% sulfur ointment available. If you were to take 1 ounce of the sulfur ointment and *add* 4 ounces of white petrolatum (0%),

   (a) What would be the percent strength of your new diluted ointment?

   (b) What would be the ratio strength of the new ointment?

**18.** How many milliliters of a 1:50 stock solution of an antiseptic are required to prepare a quart of a 1:2000 solution?

**19.** How many milliliters of water must be *added* to a pint of 95% alcohol to prepare a diluted 20% solution?

**20.** You have on hand 100 mL of concentrated dextrose injection 50%.

(a) What would be the resulting percent strength of dextrose if you *mixed* the dextrose injection with 400 mL of water for injection?

(b) How much 5% dextrose could be prepared from the dextrose injection?

(c) How much water for injection would have to be *added* to prepare the solution in item (b)?

(d) What would be the percent strength of dextrose if you *added* the concentrated dextrose to a liter bag of normal saline (0.9% NaCl)?

*The answers to all problems can be found in the **Answer Key** beginning on page 253.*

# Alligation Alternate

This section deals with a method you will not have to use very often but is a good procedure to know. This method is known as alligation alternate. Many of my students get confused at this point because they do not understand one very simple concept. The concept is that all of our previous dilutions were done with diluents that were 0% in strength. Some examples of these diluents are water, white petrolatum, and, in Question 20d, the 0.9% NaCl solution.

## *What?*

You are probably asking yourself how in the world a 0.9% NaCl solution could be 0% in strength. The "normal saline" is 0.9% sodium chloride, but it is 0% dextrose. It is also 0% sulfur, 0% borate, 0% penicillin, 0% garlic, 0% cyanide, and 0% bedbugs.

## *Get the message?*

The reason it is important to understand that we have been diluting with diluents that are 0% is because now we are going to dilute with diluents that are not 0%. I myself have used this process only a few times, because about 99% of all dilutions are simple. Now, a question before we continue.

***Question:*** If I mix 30 g of 1% hydrocortisone cream with 30 g of 2% hydrocortisone cream, I will have 60 g of a 3% hydrocortisone cream. **TRUE or FALSE?**

***Solution:*** This is absolutely **false**. You will have 60 g of a hydrocortisone cream that has a strength somewhere between 1% and 2%. In this case, 1.5% will be the strength of your new hydrocortisone mixture.

In this section, we will be using the alligation alternate method to solve dilutions made by mixing two products of known strengths to create a new product that has a percent strength somewhere between those of the two products being mixed. **Please remember** that the strength of the new product cannot be lower than the lowest percent strength you are mixing or higher than the highest percent strength.

For example, if you were to mix a 20% dextrose solution with a 5% dextrose solution, your new percent strength has to be somewhere between the strengths mixed. **The new strength cannot be more than 20% and cannot be less than 5%.** This may seem goofy, but it is a concept that many people, including some licensed professionals, do not grasp. To add insult to injury, I have met practitioners who sincerely believe that if you put twice as much 1% ointment on your skin, you will get the same results as if you'd applied a 2% ointment. That is definitely not true!

Please remember that you should use the (OV)(O%) = (NV)(N%) method when diluting with a diluent that is 0% in strength, but you should **never** use that method when diluting with two or more compounds that have a percent strength greater than 0. For this second kind of dilution, use alligation alternate.

This new technique can also be used for questions with 0% diluents, but I do not recommend using it for such problems.

In the *alligation alternate* method for diluting, you will solve for the *proportional number of parts* of each component to be mixed.

*All of the parts added together will equal the "whole" product you have made from the dilution. This probably makes absolutely no sense at this time, so hang in there and I will explain it further very soon.* **NOTE**

The following steps will help you better understand the *alligation alternate* process:

**Step 1.**  Make three vertical columns side by side.

**Step 2.**  In the column to the far left, place the percent concentrations of the components to be *mixed*; place the highest percent concentration above the lowest. It will be helpful to space these two percentages about 2 inches apart.

**Step 3.**  In the center column, place the percent concentration of the compound you wish to make. Situate this percentage between the percent concentrations of the two components to be *mixed*, even though they are in the left column.

**Step 4.**  In the column to the far right, place the numbers that reflect the *differences* in strength when you subtract the percent concentrations of the components (left column) from the desired percent concentration (center column). There are five very important things to remember:

  ❑ You need to subtract *diagonally*.
  ❑ You must disregard positive and negative signs.
  ❑ Your answers will be in *parts* and will have **no** unit value.
  ❑ The parts reflect the proportion of the components in the left column that are horizontally on line with them. They are **not** related to the component that has been subtracted.
  ❑ The total of all parts equals the amount of new product you are preparing.

**Step 5.**  Perform calculations using the basic ratio and proportion process. Remember that the *total* of **all** the parts equals the amount of the product you are trying to prepare. I am stressing this point, because you must understand this concept before you start setting up your ratio and proportion equations.

*Now that you are probably totally confused, let's take a look at some examples.*

*I promise these problems are not as hard as they sound.*
  *Follow all these steps, and you might even find them to be fun!*

**Example:**    In what proportion should a 5% ointment and a 15% ointment be mixed to prepare an 8% ointment?

**Solution:**    Because we are mixing two ointments to compound an *intermediate-* strength product, we will need to use the alligation alternate method for diluting. Carefully follow the steps we just discussed, relating them to this example.

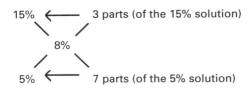

15% ⟵ 3 parts (of the 15% solution)

8%

5% ⟵ 7 parts (of the 5% solution)

**Step 1.**    Make three vertical columns.

**Step 2.**    Place percent concentrations of the components to be mixed in the left column (with 15% on top).

**Step 3.**    Place the percent concentration of the new compound (i.e., 8%) in the center.

**Step 4.**    Subtract *diagonally*, place the differences in the right column, and label these numbers as *parts*. Your answer means that you will mix **3 parts** of the **15%** ointment with **7 parts** of the **5%** ointment. After mixing these, you will have 10 parts of the new 8% ointment. Remember that the term parts just gives us a proportional value. We will place a unit value on the parts in our next example, so hang in there for a few more minutes.

**Example:**    In the previous example, how much of the 15% ointment would be required to prepare 1 lb of the 8% ointment?

**Solution:**    This may look difficult at first, but it's a piece of cake! If the *whole* amount of the 8% ointment is *10 parts* (3 parts + 7 parts), then we can say 10 parts is equal to 454 g. Now just set up a ratio and proportion calculation with 3 parts representing the 15% ointment.

10 **parts**/454 **g** = 3 **parts**/?

*136.2 g* = ?

This means you would need to use 136.2 grams of the 15% ointment.

**Question:** In the previous example, how much of the 5% ointment would be needed?

**Solution:** Again, all you need to do is a simple ratio and proportion calculation.

10 **parts**/454 **g** = 7 **parts**/?

317.8 **g** = ?

This means you would need 317.8 grams of the 5% ointment.

### Did you notice a possible shortcut?

What is the sum of all the parts? Hopefully, it is 454 grams, because we were preparing a pound of 8% ointment. Take a minute and check our answers.

| | | |
|---|---|---|
| 7 parts of 5% | = | 317.8 g |
| + 3 parts of 15% | = | 136.2 g |
| **10 parts** | | **454 g** (the total amount of 8% ointment) |

### So what is the possible shortcut?

**Answer:** If you are making 454 grams of a product and you solve for one of the two components that is going to be mixed with another component to make it, just subtract that one component from the "whole" weight of the product to find the weight of the second component. In this example, we first determined the weight of the 15% ointment to be 136.2 grams. If the total weight is going to be 454 grams, then all we need to do is subtract **454 g − 136.2 g = 317.8 g** to get the weight of the 5% ointment required to compound this product.

**Example:** From the same example, how much 8% ointment could you prepare if you had 60 grams of the 5% ointment and plenty of the 15% ointment?

**Solution:** Do a simple ratio and proportion calculation using the 5% ointment as the base since it is in limited supply. Again, the 8% ointment (i.e., the final product) is represented by "10 parts."

7 **parts**/60 **g** = 10 **parts**/?

85.7 **g** = ?

### Now you try to solve a couple of questions before we tackle the big problems!

**Question:** Continuing with the same example, how much of the 15% ointment would be mixed with 50 grams of 5% ointment to prepare the 8% ointment?

*(which I am getting very tired of!)*

**Solution:** All you need to do is say, "If 7 parts equals 50 grams, then 3 parts equals **?**"

7 **parts**/50 **g** = 3 **parts**/?

21.43 **g** = **?**

This means you would mix 21.43 grams of the 15% ointment with 50 grams of the 5% ointment to get a final weight of 71.43 grams of 8% ointment.

*Pretty cool, huh?*

**Question:** Now that you are the alligation master, let's see if you remember how to perform an *alligation medial* to check the previous question. Hopefully, you will come up with an average of **8%** for the ointment!

**Solution:** Using *alligation medial*:

| | | | | | |
|---|---|---|---|---|---|
| 50.00 g | × | 5% | = | 250.00 g% |
| 21.43 g | × | 15% | = | 321.45 g% |
| **71.43 g** | | | | **571.45 g%** |

571.45 g%/71.43 g = **8%**

## Specific Gravity

Most pharmacy practitioners rarely use specific gravity in compounding, but it is a topic you need to be aware of in case a question or a need arises. Specific gravity can be defined as the ratio (written as a decimal) of the weight of a substance to the weight of an equal volume of another substance determined to be the standard. We use water as our standard for liquids and solids. Water has a specific gravity of "1," which means that 1 mL of water weighs 1 gram (at standard temperature and pressure).

Why do you need specific gravity? Because there will be times when you will need to know the weight of a liquid or the volume of a solid, especially when you are compounding. The specific gravity of most substances can be found in pharmacy references.

## Solving Specific Gravity Problems

> *When solving for the weight of a liquid, multiply the volume in milliliters of the liquid by the specific gravity and change your answer from milliliters to grams.*

**Example:** What is the weight of a pint of chloroform (sp gr = 1.48)?

**Solution:** 480 mL × 1.48 = ***710.4 grams***

> *When solving for the volume of a substance, divide the weight of the substance in grams by the specific gravity and change your answer from grams to milliliters.*

**Example:** What is the volume of 200 g of a chemical (sp gr = 0.87)?

**Solution:** 200 g/0.87 = ***230 milliliters***

**Question:** How many kilograms would 2 liters of sorbitol (sp gr = 1.29) weigh?

**Solution:** 2000 mL × 1.29 = 2580 g = ***2.58 kilograms***

**Question:** What volume in liters would 8 lb of glycerin (sp gr = 1.25) occupy?

**Solution:** 454 g × 8 = 3632 g       3632 g/1.25 = 2906 mL = ***2.906 liters***

# PRACTICE

21. In what proportion would a 6% ointment be mixed with a 50% ointment to prepare an ointment that has a ratio strength of 1:25?

22. A 95% alcohol solution is mixed with 45% alcohol to make a 55% alcohol dilution.

    (a) In what proportions should the alcohol solutions be mixed?

    (b) How much of the 95% alcohol is required to prepare a liter of the 55% alcohol?

(c) Using your answer to item (b), how much 45% alcohol is required to prepare the mixture?

(d) How much of the 55% mixture can be prepared by mixing 45% and 95% alcohol solutions if you have only a pint of 95% alcohol and 3 gallons of 45% alcohol?

**23.** You are asked to prepare a 1:20 coal tar ointment by combining a 1:50 coal tar ointment with pure coal tar (assume 100% concentration).

(a) In what proportions should the ointment and the pure coal tar be mixed?

(b) How many grams of the 1:50 coal tar ointment will be required to prepare 1 lb of the 1:20 coal tar ointment?

(c) From your answer to item (b), how much pure coal tar will be needed?

(d) How many kilograms of the 1:20 ointment could be prepared from $\frac{1}{4}$ pound of pure coal tar (assuming an unlimited supply of the 1:50 coal tar ointment)?

**24.** For some crazy reason, you receive an order for 12% potassium chloride solution when all you have are 10% and 20% potassium chloride solutions.

(a) In what proportion would the 10% and 20% potassium chloride solutions be mixed to prepare the 12% solution?

(b) How many milliliters of 10% potassium chloride solution would be required to prepare a pint of the 12% solution?

(c) How many grams of potassium chloride would be in a pint bottle of the 12% potassium chloride solution?

(d) How many milligrams of potassium chloride would be in a tablespoonful dose of the 12% potassium chloride solution?

(e) If you only have 20% potassium chloride solution available, how many milliliters of a diluent (0% potassium chloride) would be required to prepare a liter of the 12% potassium chloride solution?

**25.** You have both 1:5 and 1:100 lidocaine HCl solutions available.

(a) Theoretically, can a 2% lidocaine HCl solution be made by mixing the two solutions?

(b) What would be the percent strength of a solution if you mixed equal volumes of the two lidocaine solutions?

(c) What would be the percent strength of a solution made by mixing the contents of a 30-mL vial of the 1:100 lidocaine with a 20-mL vial of the 1:5 lidocaine solution?

(d) Lidocaine HCl is available for IV infusion in a liter solution. The label on this solution says that it contains *0.4% lidocaine HCl in 5% dextrose*. How many milligrams of lidocaine HCl will be in 1 mL of this solution?

(e) How many grams of dextrose would a patient receive in 24 hours if she received 30 mL/hr of the solution in item (d)?

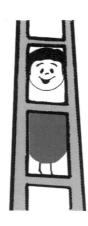

## ADVANCED PRACTICE QUESTIONS

**26.** The concentration of an antifungal agent in a cream is 1:750.

    (a) How many milligrams of the antifungal agent are in 1 gram of the cream?

    (b) What would be the percent strength of the antifungal agent in a cream prepared by mixing a 118-gram tube of the antifungal cream with 60 grams of a cream base that contains no antifungal agent?

**27.** Rx    Hydrochloric acid    10%
        disp.    30 mL
        Sig.    20 gtt in water and use as directed

    (a) How many milligrams of hydrochloric acid are in one dose given with a dispensing dropper that delivers 25 gtt/mL?

    (b) What would be the resulting percent strength of hydrochloric acid in item (a) if the prescribed volume was mixed with 1 teaspoonful of water?

**28.** Rx    Cinnamon oil in alcohol solution 1:400
        Sig.   As directed

    (a) How many liters of this prescription can be made from 35 mL of cinnamon oil?

    (b) What would be the percent strength of a solution made by adding 100 mL of alcohol to 35 mL of cinnamon oil?

29. Rx    Boric acid         500 mg
        Water q.s. ad     30 mL
        Sig.    As directed

    (a) How many milliliters of a 10% boric acid solution would be used to prepare this prescription?

    (b) What would be the ratio strength of boric acid in the final product?

30. Dextrose pediatric injection contains 2500 mg/10 mL in a prefilled syringe.

    (a) What is the percent strength of this injection?

    (b) What would be the percent strength of dextrose in a solution made by mixing one such syringe with 50 mL of D5W?

31. Diazepam is available as an oral solution (concentrate) 5 mg/mL. This concentrate is supplied in 30-mL bottles with a calibrated dropper (which has a graduation of 0.2 mL per milligram).

    (a) What is the percent strength of the concentrate?

    (b) What would be the percent strength of a solution made by diluting 0.4 mL of diazepam concentrate up to 60 mL with orange juice?

32. Cefazolin for injection USP is supplied in 500-mg single-dose vials that need to be reconstituted with 2 mL of sterile water for injection, giving an approximate available volume of 2.2 mL.

    (a) What is the approximate concentration of cefazolin in the reconstituted vial in milligrams per milliliter?

(b) For intravenous administration, dilute the reconstituted vial with 5 mL of 0.9% sodium chloride injection. What is the resulting concentration in milligrams per milliliter?

33. Filgrastim is available in single-dose, preservative-free vials containing 300 mcg (1 mL) of filgrastim (300 mcg/mL). If required, filgrastim may be diluted in 5% dextrose injection. Dilution to a final concentration of less than 5 mcg/mL is not recommended at any time.

(a) Express the minimum concentration as a percent strength.

(b) How much 5% dextrose injection is needed to dilute 1 vial to the minimum allowable concentration?

34. Ampicillin sodium/sulbactam sodium parenteral combination is available as a white to off-white dry powder for reconstitution. This antibacterial combination is available in vials containing 1.5 g (1 g ampicillin and 0.5 g sulbactam). It is also available as a 3-g vial with the same 2:1 proportion as the 1.5-g vial.

(a) How much sulbactam would be contained in a mixture of 1 vial of the 1.5-g strength and 3 vials of the 3-g strength?

(b) Vials for intramuscular use may be reconstituted with sterile water for injection USP. The 3-g vial requires 6.4 mL of diluent to be added, resulting in a final "withdrawal volume" of 8 mL. What is the percent strength of ampicillin in the reconstituted solution?

**35.** Ketoconazole cream 2% is supplied in 15-g, 30-g, and 60-g tubes.

(a) What would be the resulting percent strength of a cream prepared by combining the contents of all sizes of tubes? (This is a tough one, so be careful.)

(b) How much pure ketoconazole must be mixed with a 30-g tube of this ketaconazole cream to prepare a 1.5% ketoconazole cream?

*The answers to all problems can be found in the **Answer Key** beginning on page 253.*

# Electrolyte Solutions

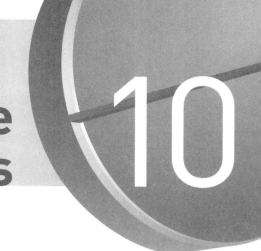

**10**

I have discovered over the years that the subject of electrolyte solutions and, more specifically, **milliequivalents**, tends to strike fear into the hearts of most students and practitioners. Fortunately, as a pharmacy technician, you will rarely have to deal with problems related to milliequivalents unless you are in a very specialized practice setting. Also, most electrolyte solutions have both the "milligram" strength and the "milliequivalent" strength printed on their labels.

Since you may have a limited background in chemistry, I will strive to follow my promise to K.I.S.S. (Please turn back to the preface if you have forgotten what this means.) And, if you happen to have a Ph.D. in chemistry, please forgive me for oversimplifying a complicated subject!

All living cells are made up of atoms and molecules. The human body not only is composed of atoms, but also runs on them. I guess you could technically say we are "atomic"-powered machines. All of us have countless atoms such as sodium, potassium, calcium, magnesium, chlorine, oxygen, and hydrogen that are constantly moving in and out of our cells and body. These atoms frequently combine with other atoms due to bonding by electrical charges, forming molecules.

**OBJECTIVES**

Upon mastery of Chapter 10 you will be able to:

- Understand the meaning and significance of electrolyte solutions.
- Recognize the valence of selected ions.
- Understand atomic weight and calculate molecular weight.
- Define a milliequivalent.
- Solve problems related to electrolyte solutions.

# Getting Molecular

Some examples of molecules are potassium chloride, dihydrogen oxide (i.e., water, also referred to as $H_2O$), and sodium chloride. Most of these molecules break apart when put into solutions, forming particles known as ions. An example is when sodium chloride (NaCl) is put into water; it dissociates (i.e., breaks apart) into sodium (Na) and chloride (Cl) ions. The sodium has a positive (+) charge, and the chloride has a negative (–) charge. Because of this, we say that ions carry an electrical charge and are **electrolytes**.

Some molecules, such as dextrose and urea, do not dissociate in body water. We refer to these molecules as **nonelectrolytes**. Both electrolytes and nonelectrolytes are critical to the operation and maintenance of the human body. When they are out of balance due to disease, dehydration, or other causes, the human body can fail to function appropriately, resulting in serious illness or even death.

Throughout this textbook, we have discussed many examples and worked numerous problems related to electrolytes and nonelectrolytes. When I mentioned potassium chloride solutions, normal saline solutions, and IVs with dextrose in water, we were actually addressing electrolyte and nonelectrolyte products.

Every day in pharmacy practice, you will fill prescriptions for replacement therapy. These prescriptions will range from tablets to liquids to intravenous solutions. Let's take a few minutes to review a little more about electrolytes, atoms, and molecules.

For your sanity and mine, I am going to limit the scope of our discussion to just a few atoms and molecules that you will encounter frequently in everyday pharmacy practice. There are many others, but we cannot cover them all, which I am sure breaks your heart!

Each atom has an atomic weight (which can be found in various textbooks). When atoms combine to form molecules, their molecular weights can be calculated by simply adding the atomic weights of the atoms in the molecule.

Here are some properties of common elements:

| Element | Formula | Atomic Weight | Valence |
| --- | --- | --- | --- |
| Aluminum | Al | 27 | +3 |
| Calcium | Ca | 40 | +2 |
| Chloride | Cl | 35.5 | −1 |
| Iron (II) | Fe | 56 | +2 |
| Hydrogen | H | 1 | +1 |
| Magnesium | Mg | 24 | +2 |
| Potassium | K | 39 | +1 |
| Sodium | Na | 23 | +1 |

There are numerous other ions that are combinations of atoms bonded tightly together. Common examples of this kind of ion are:

| Ions and Formulas | | Weight | Valence |
|---|---|---|---|
| Ammonium | $(NH_4)$ | 18 | +1 |
| Acetate | $(C_2H_3O_2)$ | 59 | −1 |
| Bicarbonate | $(HCO_3)$ | 61 | −1 |
| Carbonate | $(CO_3)$ | 60 | −2 |
| Citrate | $(C_6H_5O_7)$ | 189 | −3 |
| Gluconate | $(C_6H_{11}O_7)$ | 195 | −1 |
| Lactate | $(C_3H_5O_3)$ | 89 | −1 |
| Phosphate | $(H_2PO_4)$ | 97 | −1 |
| | $(HPO_4)$ | 96 | −2 |
| Sulfate | $(SO_4)$ | 96 | −2 |

### So, what is all this valence stuff?

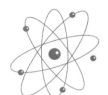

This explanation oversimplifies a complicated topic, but think of ions as magnets. Positive and negative poles attract each other, and poles that are of the same charge push each other apart. With this in mind, let's think about several molecules you are familiar with and see how their different charges interact.

**Examples:** *Sodium chloride (NaCl)* – Notice from your table that sodium has a (+1) valence (or *charge*) and chloride has a (−1) valence, so the 2 atoms combine (or *attract*), creating a molecule known as sodium chloride.

*Potassium chloride (KCl)* – Same concept as NaCl, with potassium (+1) instead of sodium.

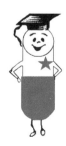

*Calcium chloride (?)* – Looking at the table, you will notice that calcium has a valence of (+2), so how many chloride ions (−1) do you think the calcium ion would attract? If you said 2, then you get a star! The molecule calcium chloride has 1 calcium ion and 2 chloride ions and is written $CaCl_2$.

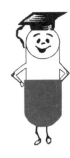

## Now you try several of these to see if you are catching on!

**Question:** How many sodium ions would be attracted to 1 sulfate ion?

**Solution:** Because the sulfate ion ($SO_4$) has a (−2) valence, it will attract 2 sodium ions and is properly written as $Na_2SO_4$.

**Question:** How many calcium ions do you think would be in calcium carbonate?

**Solution:** The calcium ion has a (+2) valence, and the carbonate ion has a (−2) valence, so only 1 ion of calcium will bind with 1 ion of carbonate to make calcium carbonate, also known as $CaCO_3$.

**Question:** How many gluconate ions are in a molecule of calcium gluconate?

**Solution:** The calcium ion has a valence of (+2), and the gluconate ion has a valence of (−1), so the calcium ion will attract 2 gluconate ions. The molecular structure will look like this: $Ca(C_6H_{11}O_7)_2$, or $C_{12}H_{22}CaO_{14}$.

**Question:** What is the structure of aluminum chloride?

**Solution:** Because the aluminum ion has a valence of (+3), it will attract 3 chloride ions (−1). The molecular structure will be $AlCl_3$.

**Question:** What is the structure of magnesium sulfate?

**Solution:** Because a magnesium ion has a valence of (+2) and a sulfate ion has a valence of (−2), 1 ion of each will attract. The molecular structure will be $MgSO_4$.

*In some products, you will have the hydrated form of chemicals, which means the molecules will have water molecules ($H_2O$) attached. (Examples would be $CaCl_2 \cdot 2H_2O$ and $MgSO_4 \cdot 7H_2O$.) I think this is going beyond the information you need for everyday practice, but it is important to know if there are waters of hydration attached to a molecule. If there are, you **MUST** count the water molecules as part of the molecular weight of the overall molecule when solving for milliequivalents.*

# Milliequivalents (mEq)

The concentration of electrolytes in a solution is frequently expressed in units known as milliequivalents (abbreviated mEq). A milliequivalent is a unit of measurement of the amount of chemical activity of an electrolyte. Again, I am oversimplifying this concept to make it easier for you to understand.

Please refer to a chemistry textbook if you have a burning desire for more detail and scientific explanations or if I have insulted your intelligence. This chapter should adequately prepare you for most mEq problems without your having to search far and wide for more stimulating explanations!

*What in the world is a milliequivalent, and how can it be measured?*

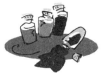

Electrolytes and nonelectrolytes normally are ordered by the physician in either *milligrams* or *milliequivalents.* I think the best way to explain milliequivalents is by relating them directly to milligrams, which you are already familiar with.

**Step 1.** Calculate the atomic weight (AW) or molecular weight (MW) of an element and consider the weight to be in milligrams. *Example*: sodium = 23 mg and chloride = 35.5 mg, so the weight of sodium chloride would be 23 mg + 35.5 mg = **58.5 mg.**

*This is not the actual weight of a molecule of sodium chloride. It is actually the weight of a millimole of sodium chloride, but that is another complicated story for another time!*

**Step 2.** Now take the atomic or molecular weight (expressed in milligrams) and *divide* that number by the **highest** valence of its two ions (disregard the positive or negative signs).

*Let's look at several examples, since this has probably totally confused you!*

***Example:*** How many milligrams are in a milliequivalent of sodium?

**Step 1.** The atomic weight of sodium is 23 (call this 23 mg).

**Step 2.** Since sodium has a valence of +1, divide 23 mg by 1. There are 23 mg of sodium in a mEq of sodium (i.e., 23 mg/1 = 23 mg).

***Example:*** How many milligrams are in a milliequivalent of calcium?

**Step 1.** The atomic weight of calcium is 40 (call this 40 mg).

**Step 2.** Since calcium has a valence of +2, divide 40 mg by 2. There are 20 mg of calcium in a mEq of calcium (i.e., 40 mg/2 = 20 mg).

*Example:*    How many milligrams are in a milliequivalent of potassium chloride?

Step 1.    The molecular weight of KCl is 39 + 35.5 = **74.5 mg.**

Step 2.    Since the two valences are +1 and −1, disregard the sign and just divide 74.5 mg by 1. This means there are 74.5 mg of potassium chloride in a milliequivalent of KCl (i.e., 74.5 mg/1 = 74.5 mg).

*Example:*    How many milligrams are in a milliequivalent of calcium chloride?

Step 1.    The molecular weight of $CaCl_2$ is 111. This problem is a little different from the previous examples, because there are 2 chloride ions and 1 calcium ion (35.5 + 35.5 + 40 = **111 mg**).

Step 2.    The chloride ions have a valence of −1, and the calcium has a valence of +2. Divide 111 mg by 2 (i.e., the largest valence regardless of sign). There are 55.5 mg in a mEq of $CaCl_2$ (i.e., 111 mg/2 = 55.5 mg).

> As mentioned earlier, if calcium chloride is in the hydrated form, it will have the structure $CaCl_2 \cdot 2H_2O$, and its molecular weight will be 147 instead. A milliequivalent of hydrated calcium chloride will be 147 mg/2 = 73.5 mg.

*Example:*    How many milligrams are in a milliequivalent of potassium citrate?

Step 1.    The molecular weight of $C_6H_5K_3O_7$ is 306.
Citrate $(C_6H_5O_7)$ = 189 mg and 3 potassiums = 3 × 39 mg = **117 mg** for a total molecular weight of 117 mg + 189 mg = **306 mg.**

Step 2.    The 3 potassium ions each have a valence of +1, and the citrate ion has a valence of −3. Divide 306 mg by 3 (i.e., the largest valence regardless of sign). There are 102 mg in a mEq of potassium citrate (i.e., 306 mg/3 = 102 mg).

**Remember this concept:** Whenever you have a milliequivalent of any compound, you can make a statement of unity: "1 milliequivalent of the molecule yields upon dissociation 1 mEq of each of the ions that made up the original molecule."

*Example:*    In the last example, we determined that there are 102 mg of potassium citrate per milliequivalent of potassium citrate. We can say that **1** mEq of *potassium citrate* (i.e., 102 mg) yields upon dissociation **1** mEq of *potassium* ion and **1** mEq of *citrate* ion.

*Now I realize this might not make a lot of sense, but trust me on this one, because it is getting late and I am hungry!*

*How can you use this statement of unity in practice?*

**Example:**   How much potassium citrate would provide 5 mEq of potassium?

**Solution:**   Based on our *statement of unity* just discussed, **1** mEq of potassium is contained in **1** mEq of potassium citrate. By using basic logic, we know that **5** mEq of potassium would be contained in **5** mEq of potassium citrate. Now, by using the ratio and proportion process, solve for the answer in milligrams. Remember from the last example that there were 102 mg of potassium citrate per milliequivalent.

102 **mg K-citrate**/1 **mEq K-citrate** = ?/5 **mEq K-citrate**

510 **mg potassium citrate** = ?

*This means that you would give the patient 510 mg of potassium citrate, which is the same as giving 5 mEq of potassium citrate or 5 mEq of potassium, which is just what the doctor ordered!*

*Now it is your turn to try a tough one!*

**Question:**   What would be the percent strength of a sodium bicarbonate injection if the label on its vial read "0.9 mEq sodium bicarbonate per milliliter"?

**Solution:**

**Step 1.**   The molecular weight of sodium bicarbonate equals 84.

**Step 2.**   84 mg/1 = 84 mg sodium bicarbonate per mEq of sodium bicarbonate.

*To solve for percent strength, just convert (mEq/mL) to (mg/mL) to (grams/100 mL).*

1 **mEq sod. bicarb.**/84 **mg sod. bicarb.** = 0.9 **mEq sod. bicarb.**/?

75.6 **mg sodium bicarbonate** = ?

This means there are 75.6 mg of sodium bicarbonate per mL, **or** 7560 mg/100 mL: 7560 mg/100 mL → 7.56 g/100 mL → ***7.56% solution of sodium bicarbonate.***

# PRACTICE

1. A patient has a prescription for one pint of 10% potassium chloride liquid.

   (a) How many grams of potassium chloride (KCl) are in the bottle?

   (b) How many milliequivalents of potassium chloride are in the bottle?

   (c) How many mEq of *potassium* are in the bottle?

   (d) How many mEq of potassium chloride are in a tablespoonful dose of this solution?

   (e) How many milliliters of this solution would a patient receive daily if her physician orders 10 mEq of *potassium* q.i.d.?

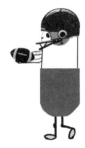

2. A professional football player takes 1-gram sodium chloride (NaCl) tablets during the hot summer days in football camp.

   (a) How many milliequivalents of sodium chloride are in each tablet?

   (b) How many mEq of *sodium* does the football player receive from these tablets in a week if he takes 1 tablet t.i.d.?

   (c) If his trainer wants him to receive 100 mEq of *sodium* each day, how many tablets should he take?

3. How many grams of sodium chloride are required to prepare a liter of a solution containing 154 mEq of sodium chloride?

4. What is the percent strength of the solution in question 3?

5. A physician likes to write orders for patients to receive 1 mEq of *sodium* per kilogram of body weight.

   (a) How many milligrams of sodium chloride would a 72-kg patient receive?

   (b) How many grams of sodium chloride would a 110-pound patient receive?

   (c) How much normal saline (0.9% NaCl) would provide the sodium chloride for the patient in item (b)?

   (d) How many milliliters of concentrated 14.6% sodium chloride injection would provide the sodium for the patient in item (b)?

6. If a patient receives 100 mL of 5% dextrose and normal saline ($D_5NS$) every hour, how many milliequivalents of *sodium* will she receive in 24 hours?

7. You receive an order to prepare a solution containing 30 mEq of calcium per liter.

   (a) How many milligrams of calcium chloride ($CaCl_2$) are required to prepare this solution? (Let's use MW = 111.)

   (b) What is the percent concentration of calcium chloride in this solution?

8. You are asked to prepare a solution of sodium bicarbonate to contain 90 mEq of *sodium* per 100 mL.

   (a) How many milligrams of sodium bicarbonate ($NaHCO_3$) is needed to prepare a liter of this solution?

   (b) What is the percent concentration of sodium bicarbonate in this solution?

9. The directions on a vial of ammonium chloride say to add a 20-mL vial of ammonium chloride containing 100 mEq of ammonium chloride to 500 mL of normal saline.

   (a) What is the percent strength of ammonium chloride ($NH_4Cl$) in the vial?

   (b) What is the percent strength of ammonium chloride when added to the 500 mL of normal saline?

10. Sodium acetate injection is available in 50-mL vials containing 4 mEq/mL.

    (a) How many milliliters of this injection would provide a 1-gram dose?

Sodium acetate = $NaC_2H_3O_2$    MW = 82    Valence = 1

    (b) How many milliequivalents of *sodium* are in 5 mL of this injection?

    (c) What is the percent strength of sodium acetate in this solution?

## ADVANCED PRACTICE QUESTIONS

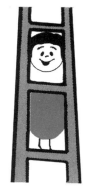

**11.** Infant 4.2% sodium bicarbonate injection is available as a 10-mL unit-of-use syringe and contains 0.5 mEq/mL.

(a) How many milligrams of sodium bicarbonate are in the syringe?

(b) How many milliequivalents of sodium bicarbonate are in the syringe?

(c) Without looking back in your book, how many milligrams would you estimate 1 mEq of sodium bicarbonate weighs?

(d) What would be the percent strength of a sodium bicarbonate solution that contained 2.5 mEq/mL?

**12.** Rx    Potassium chloride solution (0.8 mEq/mL)
         disp.    1 pint

(a) How many grams of potassium chloride will be required to prepare this prescription? (MW KCl = 74.5)

(b) What is the percent strength of this solution?

**13.** Rx    Calcium chloride solution 5%
         disp.    240 mL
         sig.    1 teaspoonful    q.i.d.

(a) How many milliequivalents of calcium chloride will the patient receive daily? (MW calcium chloride = 111) (valence of calcium = +2)

(b) How many milliequivalents of calcium are in the entire prescription?

**14.** A 20-mL ampule of sterile potassium chloride solution contains 2 mEq/mL.

(a) What is the percent strength of the solution? (MW of potassium chloride = 74.5)

(b) What is the percent strength of a solution made by diluting the contents of one such ampule to a liter with sterile water?

**15.** Phenytoin sodium injection USP is a sterile solution containing in each milliliter 50 mg of phenytoin sodium. ($C_{15}H_{11}N_2NaO_2$   MW = 274) ($Na^+$   AW = 23)

(a) How many grams of phenytoin sodium are in a 6-mL dose of this injection?

(b) Approximately how many milliequivalents of sodium will a patient receive if the dose in item (a) is given daily for 3 days?

**16.** Sodium bicarbonate is available in 50-mEq/50-mL prefilled syringes. ($NaHCO_3$   MW = 84) ($Na^+$ AW = 23)

(a) How many milligrams of sodium bicarbonate are in each milliliter of the solution?

(b) What is the percent strength of sodium bicarbonate in the solution?

(c) How many milliequivalents of sodium are in a syringe?

(d) How many milliequivalents of bicarbonate are in a milliliter of the solution?

**17.** Calcium gluconate injection is available as a 10% solution.
($C_{12}H_{22}CaO_{14}$   MW = 430) ($Ca^{++}$ MW = 40)

(a) The normal adult dose of this injection is 500 mg to 2 g. How many milliliters will provide the maximum dose?

(b) What would be the percent strength of calcium gluconate if you diluted a 10-mL bottle of this calcium gluconate injection with 100 mL of a 0.9% sodium chloride solution?

(c) How many milliequivalents of calcium ion are in a 50-mL vial of this calcium gluconate injection?

(d) The dose of this calcium gluconate injection for a pediatric patient is 2 to 5 mL. How many milliequivalents of calcium ion are in the lower dose?

*The answers to all problems can be found in the **Answer Key** beginning on page 253.*

# Temperature Conversions

In 1709, Gabriel D. Fahrenheit, a German physicist, invented an alcohol thermometer. Seven years later, he improved his thermometer by using mercury instead of alcohol. The scale he used on the improved thermometer indicated that (at sea level) water started to freeze at 32° and water started to boil at 212°. This was the beginning of the Fahrenheit scale for measuring temperature. This scale has been used in many parts of the world for centuries, and it is the primary measure of temperature used in the United States.

Several decades after Fahrenheit's scale was established, a Swedish astronomer named Anders Celsius suggested a more convenient thermometer based on water starting to freeze at 0° and starting to boil at 100°. We are now faced with the reality that when measuring temperature, some people use the Fahrenheit (°F) scale and others use the Celsius or centigrade (°C) scale. (Does this sound a lot like our chapter on "conversions"?) For your sanity and mine, I am going to make this a really short chapter (sweet and simple)! All you really need to know is how to convert back and forth between the two scales.

There are two or three formulas commonly used for converting between the Fahrenheit and centigrade (Celsius) systems. You may be familiar with some that use fractions such as $\frac{9}{5}$, $\frac{5}{9}$, and 0.55. For the sake of simplicity, I want you to learn only what I consider the easiest and least confusing formulas and to forget about those "common" fractions.

## OBJECTIVES

Upon mastery of Chapter 11 you will be able to:

- Explain the differences between the Fahrenheit and centigrade scales.
- Convert degrees centigrade to degrees Fahrenheit.
- Convert degrees Fahrenheit to degrees centigrade.

## The How-to Stuff

*To convert from centigrade to Fahrenheit:*    °F = (1.8 × °C) + 32

*To convert from Fahrenheit to centigrade:*    °C = (°F − 32) ÷ 1.8

**Example:**    Convert 100°C (the boiling point of water) to degrees Fahrenheit.

*You should already know this answer based on our previous discussion, but let's try it and see if our formula really works.*

**Solution:**    °F = (1.8 × °C) + 32
°F = (1.8 × 100°) + 32
°F = (180°) + 32
°F = **212°**

**Example:**    Do you remember at what centigrade temperature water freezes? If you do not remember, I'll give you a hint: at 32°F. Now, plug this information into your other formula, and see if the formula works.

**Solution:**    °C = (°F − 32) ÷ 1.8
°C = (32° − 32) ÷ 1.8
°C = (0°) ÷ 1.8
°C = **0°**

*Now you try to solve a couple of these questions.*

**Question:**    A baby's rectal temperature is measured with a thermometer to be 102°F. Express this temperature in degrees centigrade.

**Solution:**    °C = (°F − 32) ÷ 1.8
°C = (102° − 32) ÷ 1.8
°C = (70°) ÷ 1.8
°C = **38.9°**

**Question:**    Would you put on a sweater if the temperature sign at your neighborhood bank said it was 49°C?

**Solution:**    °F = (1.8 × °C) + 32
°F = (1.8 × 49°) + 32
°F = (88.2°) + 32
°F = **120.2°**

*I hope you do not need a sweater!*

# PRACTICE

**1.** Convert the following Fahrenheit temperatures to degrees centigrade.

(a) 41°F

(b) 86°F

(c) 167°F

(d) 14°F

(e) −40°F

**2.** Convert the following centigrade temperatures to degrees Fahrenheit.

(a) 15°C

(b) 75°C

(c) 0°C

(d) −5°C

(e) −75°C

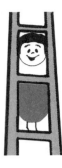

## ADVANCED PRACTICE QUESTIONS

3.  The temperature this past winter reached –20°C. Express this temperature in degrees Fahrenheit.

4.  A solution freezes at 23°F. Express this temperature in degrees centigrade.

5.  Certain crystals melt at 60°C. Express this temperature in degrees Fahrenheit.

6.  The temperature inside a car exposed to full sunlight can rise above 177°F. Express this temperature in degrees centigrade.

7.  A type of rubber can crack at –15°C. Express this temperature in degrees Fahrenheit.

8.  The temperature in Alaska dipped to –58°F. Express this temperature in degrees centigrade.

9.  An oil melts at 30°C, which would be equivalent to _____ degrees Fahrenheit.

10. Insulin should be stored at 40°F, which would be equivalent to _____ degrees centigrade.

**11.** An aerosol freezes at −111°C. Express this temperature in degrees Fahrenheit.

**12.** The normal oral temperature for an adult is 98.6°F. Express this temperature in degrees centigrade.

**13.** Filgrastim is a human granulocyte colony-stimulating factor and is available in single-dose, preservative-free vials that should be stored at 2°C to 8°C.

   (a) Express this temperature range in °F.

   (b) Where should this product be stored?

**14.** Ketorolac tromethamine injection USP needs to be stored at 68°F to 77°F.

   (a) Express this temperature range in °C.

   (b) Where should this product be stored?

**15.** Nesiritide is provided as a sterile lyophilized powder in 1.5-mg single-use vials. The label states that it should be stored below 25°C and not frozen. Express this approximate storage range in °F.

*The answers to all problems can be found in the **Answer Key** beginning on page 253.*

# Business Math

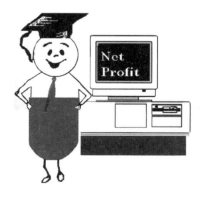

W e are coming down the "home stretch," but even though you are the master of practically everything you need to know about pharmacy math, you still need to learn about the marketing or business aspects of pharmacy practice. Every pharmacy you work in is likely to have its own approach to pricing and discounting, and there are many variations on business math. In this chapter, we will look at basic terms and procedures so that you will be able to function in the "business" world of pharmacy.

## Common Business Terms

*Here are some basic business terms you ought to know:*

**AWP** – (*Average Wholesale Price*) The published "theoretical" price a pharmacy pays for a medication (theoretical because pharmacies normally pay less than the AWP due to discounts, contracts with wholesalers, special deals, group purchasing, etc).

**Markup** – The difference between the cost and the selling price of an item of merchandise.

**Gross margin** – (also referred to as *gross profit*) This is the difference between the selling price and the acquisition (purchase) price; usually refers to the total inventory.

**Overhead** – The expenses associated with doing business, such as rent, utilities, and salaries.

**Net profit** – The true profit after all associated expenses are subtracted (i.e., the gross profit minus overhead expenses).

**Markdown** – (also referred to as a *discount* or a *sale*) A reduction of a set price.

**Inventory** – An itemized list of the merchandise and its cost in a particular establishment.

**Turnover rate** – How often an establishment's total inventory is sold over a specific time period.

## Markup

*Markup* is a term that is often used interchangeably with gross margin and gross profit. If you purchase a television set from a local retailer for $189 and the retailer paid $150 to the manufacturer for the television, then the retailer's *markup* is $39.

$$\textbf{Markup} = \textbf{selling price} - \textbf{cost}$$

**$39** = $189 − $150

*Question:*    What would be the markup on an antibiotic a pharmacy purchased from a wholesaler for $25 and sold to a patient for $32?

*Solution:*    **Markup = selling price − cost**

**$7** = $32 − $25

## Percent Markup

*Percent markup* (*percent of gross margin*) is the percentage determined by dividing the markup by the **selling price** or, in some cases, by the **cost** of the merchandise. It is very important for you to clarify what the *percent markup* is based on. Let's use the last example to determine the percent markup both by *selling price* and by *cost*.

**Percent markup = (selling price − cost)/*selling price***
(*based on **selling price***)

= ($32 − $25)/$32

= $7/$32 = 0.219 = **21.9%** percent markup (based on ***selling price***)

## Percent markup = (selling price − cost)/*cost*
(*based on **cost***)

$$= (\$32 - \$25)/\$25$$

$$= \$7/\$25 = 0.28 = \textbf{28\%} \text{ percent markup (based on } \textbf{\textit{cost}})$$

**Question:** What is the percent markup based on *selling price* of a laxative that cost the pharmacy $3.50 and is sold to a patient for $5.50?

**Solution:** % markup = ($5.50 − $3.50)/$5.50

% markup = $2.00/$5.50 = 0.36 = **36%** markup (based on selling price)

**Question:** In the previous question, what is the percent markup based on *cost*?

**Solution:** % markup = ($5.50 − $3.50)/$3.50

% markup = $2.00/$3.50 = **57%** markup
(based on cost)

**Question:** A pharmacy purchases a sunscreen from a wholesaler for $5. The store's policy is to mark up all nonprescription products 45% based on *cost*. What will be the selling price after the markup?

**Solution:** You are going to have to think about this problem a little bit before calculating. Some people like to solve for 45% of $5, which is $2.25, and then add the numbers together to get a selling price of **$7.25**. I like to simply multiply the cost ($5) times a factor of 1.45 (i.e., 145%) to get $7.25.

**Question:** Using the last example, what would be the price if the store's policy was to mark up all nonprescription products by 45% based on the *selling price*?

**Solution:** *Please note that this problem is worked differently than the previous one.* If the markup is 45% of the selling price, then the cost would be 55% of that price (100% − 45% = 55%). Again, you can solve the problem by the ratio and proportion process.

55%/100% = $5/**?**

**$9.09** = ?

You can see that there is a big difference in the final cost to a consumer depending on whether the 45% fee is based on **cost** or on **selling price**.

## Percent Discounts

*Percent discounts (markdowns or sales)* occur when there is a reduction in the original selling price of an item. (Discounts also can be given by the wholesaler when a pharmacy pays its bills within a certain time frame.) These discounts are almost always based on *selling price* and can be solved in a similar manner to our last example, which was also based on *selling price*.

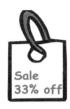

**Example:** Let's pretend you go to the mall for an after-holiday sale and see an $80 outfit on sale for 33% off the ticketed price. How much would the outfit cost after the discount?

**Solution:** If 100% of the price is $80, then you will only have to pay 67%. In other words, 100% original price − 33% discount = 67%.

67%/100% = **?**/$80

$53.60 = **?**

**Question:** The pharmacy you work at is selling humidifiers for 25% off. What would a humidifier originally priced at $35 cost after the markdown is taken off?

**Solution:** Consider the original price, $35, to be 100%. The price after the sale is 75% of the original price (100% − 25% = 75%).

100%/75% = $35/**?**

$26.25 = **?**

## Gross Profit

Although *gross profit (gross margin)* is similar to markup, it typically is used to refer more to the big picture of store sales. In contrast, markup is generally associated with individual products. *Gross profit* is the difference between total sales minus the cost of the items sold.

**Example:** If a store has sales totaling $2,000,000 and the cost of the items sold was $1,500,000, then the *gross profit* is $500,000 (i.e., sales − cost = gross profit).

# Net Profit

*Net profit* is what some people affectionately call the bottom line. It is the true profit that store owners are concerned with. The difference between *net* profit and *gross* profit is that *net profit* subtracts from total sales **both** the cost of goods sold **and** the store's overhead expenses.

**Example:**    Using the previous example for gross profit, what is the net profit if the store's overhead expenses (i.e., security, rent, electricity, insurance, and technicians' *high* salaries) total about $350,000?

**Solution:**    Net profit = sales − (cost of goods + overhead)

Net profit = $2,000,000 − ($1,500,000 + $350,000)

Net profit = $2,000,000 − $1,850,000

Net profit = $150,000

As mentioned earlier, gross and net profits can be used to analyze annual sales, monthly sales, and even the sale of a single prescription. Also, many store owners study various departments within a store (cosmetics, durable medical equipment, nonprescription drugs, etc.) to establish which areas produce the best profits and which are performing poorly.

# Inventory Turnover Rate

Most pharmacies take an *inventory* (a count of all store items and their costs) at least once a year. Inventory *turnover* is the frequency with which items sell over a specific period. The *inventory turnover rate* can be determined by taking the cost of **all** goods purchased during a period of time and dividing this number by the average cost of the pharmacy inventory.

**Example:**    During the past 12 months, a pharmacy spent $1,800,000 on inventory purchases. Average inventory value during the past year was determined to be $300,000. What was the *inventory turnover rate*?

**Solution:**    Inventory turnover rate = total purchases/average inventory value

Inventory turnover rate = $1,800,000/$300,000 = **6 times**

*The more turnovers of inventory a store has, the better. High turnover rates indicate that the store is not investing too much money in inventory that is just sitting on the shelf looking pretty, depreciating, and possibly going out of date.*

## PRACTICE

1. A patient buys for $78 a pair of crutches that the pharmacy purchased from a durable medical equipment supplier for $45.

   (a) What is the markup on the crutches?

   (b) What is the percent markup on the crutches based on selling price?

   (c) What is the percent markup on the crutches based on cost?

   (d) What would be the price of a pair of crutches if the supplier's price remained the same but the store owner decided to charge a 72% markup based on cost?

   (e) Considering the scenario in item (d) what would be the new price if the 72% markup was based on the selling price?

2. The markup on 60 antidepressant tablets is $12, and a patient pays $78 for the entire prescription.

   (a) What was the acquisition cost of the tablets for the pharmacy?

   (b) What was the average cost to the patient for each tablet?

   (c) What was the markup on each tablet?

(d) If the patient takes 1 tablet b.i.d., what will the cost be to the patient for a week of antidepressant therapy?

(e) What was the percent markup on the prescription based on cost?

(f) What was the percent markup based on selling price?

3. A pharmacy accountant reported this information after an annual inventory:

Total annual overhead expenses = $850,000
Total inventory purchases = $2,670,000
Total sales = $4,300,000
Average inventory = $520,000

(a) What was the gross profit for this store?

(b) What was the net profit for this store?

(c) If the owner decided to give her pharmacy technician 5% of the net profit, how much would this be, and would you accept it?

(d) What was the inventory turnover rate?

(e) Approximately how many sales took place if the average sale was $62?

4. The prescription department had the following monthly sales information:

Net profit = $5328
Total sales receipts = $81,435
Total drug costs = $69,887

(a) What was the gross profit for the month?

(b) What was the overhead for the month?

5. A 100-tablet bottle of a new cardiovascular drug cost the pharmacy $331.

(a) With a 20% markup based on acquisition cost, how much would 30 tablets cost a patient?

(b) With a 10% markup based on selling price, how much would 60 tablets cost a patient?

(c) The wholesaler gives the pharmacy an 8% discount if all debts are paid in full in 30 days. How much would the bottle of 100 tablets cost if the pharmacy qualified for the discount?

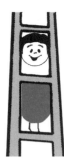

**ADVANCED PRACTICE QUESTIONS**

6. A pharmacist purchases a box of a dozen tubes of zinc oxide ointment for $14.88.

(a) What is the markup if a tube of the ointment sells for $2.69?

(b) What is the percent markup based on a selling price of $2.69?

(c)  If the product sells for $2.69, what is the percent markup based on cost?

(d)  What will a tube cost if the store offers a 30% discount on all topical products?

(e)  How much will three tubes cost if there is a 185% markup based on cost?

**7.** A pharmacy sells a bottle of 30 tablets for $38.35 and has a gross profit of 40% based on cost.

(a)  What was the original cost of the bottle of tablets?

(b)  What was the markup on each tablet?

**8.** A pharmacy purchases a gallon of potassium chloride elixir and receives a 40% discount from the wholesaler on the original price of $27.85. What is the cost of one pint of potassium chloride elixir after the discount?

**9.** A pharmacy purchases a dozen 10-dose vials of flu vaccine for $1068. How much should be charged for each vaccination to recognize a $16 profit per injection?

Flu Shots

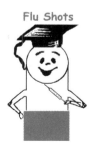

**10.**  A hospital pays $46.50 for a 20-mg vial of a drug. What would be the daily cost of the drug for a woman weighing 110 pounds if she receives 0.2 mg/kg/day?

**11.** Cremers Discount Pharmacy pays $115.85 after a 7% wholesale discount for a 100-tablet bottle of Abbadex.

   (a)  A patient named Beckett K. takes 1 Abbadex tablet t.i.d. × 10 days. How much did the pharmacy pay for Beckett's medication?

   (b)  How much would 60 tablets cost the pharmacy without the wholesale discount?

**12.** Keating Corner Drugs purchases five 60-tablet bottles of nadsopium mesylate for $305 after wholesale discounts.

   (a)  How much did the pharmacy pay for each nadsopium mesylate tablet?

   (b)  How much will it cost the pharmacy to fill a prescription for nadsopium for a pediatric patient named Kai if the prescription reads "ii tablets b.i.d. × 1 week"?

   (c)  How much profit will the pharmacy make if it dispenses Kai's prescription and Kai's insurance company reimburses the pharmacy at (cost + 4% + $3.00 dispensing fee)?

*The answers to all problems can be found in the **Answer Key** beginning on page 253.*

# Medication Errors and Clinical Challenges

13

I saved the most important information for this final chapter. If you are superstitious, I'm sorry for discussing medication errors in Chapter 13. Throughout your pharmacy career, you will hear war stories about medical and medication errors. Estimates abound regarding the number of patients killed or injured as a result of preventable mistakes by physicians, nurses, pharmacists, and even pharmacy technicians. A report by the Institute of Medicine indicated that 44,000 to 98,000 patients die annually due to these errors, making these errors the 8th leading cause of death in the United States. More people die annually from these errors than from motor vehicle accidents, breast cancer, or even AIDS. This means that 120–269 people die every day from these mistakes, which is equivalent to a medium-sized passenger plane crashing every 12 hours. I don't believe the airline industry or the FAA would find this acceptable ... do you?

So, what can you do as a pharmacy technician to prevent these errors? I sincerely believe that the first step is to be confident that you **can** make a difference. You need to be vigilant and not afraid to speak up whenever you suspect a problem may exist. I appreciate knowing I have a technician double-checking my work, and I believe most pharmacists share these feelings. So be careful, and dare to make a difference.

## OBJECTIVES

Upon mastery of Chapter 13 you will be able to:

- Understand the importance of minimizing medication errors.
- Appreciate the need for constant vigilance to avoid compounding errors.

## What Is a Medication Error?

A medication error is any preventable action or omission that may contribute to the inappropriate or harmful use of a medicine by a health professional, patient, or caregiver.

## Examples of Medication Errors

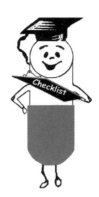

**Wrong drug** (a phone order for Xanax® is interpreted and filled as Zantac®)

**Wrong patient** (the patient in room 234 receives the medication for the patient in room 243)

**Wrong dose** (a child receives an adult dose of a medication)

**Drug allergies** (a patient allergic to sulfur receives a sulfur-containing medication)

**Contraindications** (a patient with severe liver disease receives a drug toxic to the liver)

**Wrong route** (a drug is given intramuscularly when it should be given intravenously)

**Wrong frequency** (a medication that should be given once daily is given every 6 hours)

**Equipment malfunctions** (an IV pump has a mechanical failure)

**Wrong indication** (the drug administered is inappropriate for the specific disease state)

**Calculation mistakes!!!** (no examples needed)

## Why Do Medication Errors Occur?

The list of reasons why errors occur is endless, but I believe the primary cause of medication errors is a lack of focus and concentration. In a busy pharmacy, you have constant distractions and interruptions. In addition, careless habits such as illegibly written prescriptions and medication orders can lead to disaster.

In Chapter 4, we studied a list of abbreviations commonly seen in pharmacy and medical practice. In recent years, the Joint Commission, as the primary accrediting body for healthcare providers (such as hospitals, home health care services, and nursing homes), has created a "do not use" list of common abbreviations that frequently have led to medication errors. On the next page are several examples of such abbreviations and potential problems associated with their use.

Additional information about errors can be found in the Appendix.

# Problem Abbreviations

| Abbreviation | Potential Problem | Preferred Term |
| --- | --- | --- |
| U (for unit) | Mistaken as zero, 4, or cc | Write "unit" |
| IU (for International Units) | Mistaken as IV or 10 | Write "International Units" |
| q.d. and q.o.d. | Mistaken for q.i.d. | Write "daily" or "every other day" |
| Trailing zero (3.0 mg) | Mistaken as 30 mg | Never write an unnecessary decimal point or trailing zero |
| Lack of leading zero (.3 mg) | Mistaken as 3 mg | Use a zero before a decimal point |
| MS, MSO$_4$, MgSO$_4$ | Confused for one another | Write out the words (morphine sulfate or magnesium sulfate) |
| μg (for microgram) | Mistaken for mg (milligram) | Write "mcg" |
| qHS (at bedtime) | Mistaken for "half strength" and "every hour" | Write out "half strength" or "take at bedtime" |
| t.i.w. (3 times a week) | Mistaken for 3 times a day | Write "3 times weekly" |
| SC or SQ (subcutaneous) | Mistaken as SL (sublingual) | Write "subcutaneously" |
| D/C (discharge) | Interpreted as "discontinue" | Write "discharge" |
| a.s., a.d., a.u. (left, right, or both ears) | Mistaken for o.s., o.d., o.u. (left, right, or both eyes) | Write "left ear," "right ear," or "both ears" |

## Clinical Challenges

In this final chapter, all questions are considered **"Advanced Practice."** These questions are intended to challenge your critical thinking skills and to test your ability to recognize the typical medication calculation errors that are sometimes made by nurses, pharmacists, and physicians. Use this exercise to test your skills and see if you can be 100% correct. Please try not to contribute to a disaster. **Good Luck!**

1. Rx    Ceclor® 500 mg

   How many milliliters of a 375-mg/5-mL Ceclor oral suspension would provide the prescribed dose?

2. A patient is to receive 62.5 mcg of benztropine mesylate. How many 0.5-mg tablets would provide the prescribed dose?

3. A patient is to receive gentamicin 100 mg IM. How much of an 80-mg/2-mL solution should be used?

4. A patient is to receive 60 mEq of Kaon® daily in four divided doses. How much of a 20-mEq/15-mL Kaon solution should be given every 6 hours?

5. A patient is to receive 2 g daily of dicloxacillin sodium in four divided doses. How many milliliters of a 62.5-mg/teaspoonful suspension would provide a single dose?

6. A patient is to receive 75 mcg IV of fentanyl. How much of a 0.05-mg/mL solution is needed?

**7.** A patient is to receive a liter of normal saline over 7 hours. How many drops per minute are required to administer the normal saline if the IV set has a drip factor of 10 gtt/mL?

**8.** A physician writes an order for Vistaril® 25 mg and Demerol® 25 mg IM. Demerol is available in 1-mL ampules in a 50-mg/mL strength, and Vistaril is available in a 25-mg/mL strength. What is the total volume that must be injected to provide the prescribed dose?

**9.** A nurse hangs an IVPB containing 500 mg of an antibiotic. The volume is 100 mL, and the pharmacy sends instructions to run the IV over 30 minutes. For how many milliliters per hour should the IV pump be set?

**10.** A physician orders 90 mL of 10% dextrose to infuse at 50 gtt/minute. How many minutes will it take for the solution to infuse using an IV set that delivers 15 gtt/mL?

**11.** A 250-mL IV is started at 1900 hours and is set to run at 30-mL/hour. When will the infusion run out?

**12.** A 500-mL D5W bag contains 25,000 units of heparin, and the IV is set to deliver 20 mL/hr. How many units of heparin will the patient receive each hour?

**13.** A patient is to receive lidocaine 2 g in 250 mL D5W at a rate of 2 mg/minute. At what flow rate will this medication be infused?

14. Nitroglycerin is infusing at 8 mL/hour. The IV bag contains 50 mg of nitro-glycerin in 250 mL of D5W. How many micrograms per minute is the patient receiving?

15. A patient is to receive 100 mL of albumin 5% over 2 hours. What will be the IV's flow rate in milliliters per minute?

16. An infant is on fluid restriction and is limited to 50 mL of formula every 4 hours. The baby also receives a medication every 6 hours that is diluted in a fluid ounce of water. What is the infant's 24-hour fluid intake?

17. An order is received for penicillin G potassium. The patient is to receive 2.5 million units IV q.6h. This antibiotic is available in 1,000,000-unit vials. The instructions on the vial indicate to add 1.6 mL of diluent, which will yield a concentration of 500,000 units/mL. How many milliliters will provide the appropriate dose?

18. A child is to receive 60 mg of gentamicin. The pharmacy prepares this medication as a 50-mL piggyback. According to the package insert, genta-micin can be delivered at a rate of 1–2 mg/minute. What is the recommended time range over which this medication should be administered?

19. A 55-lb child is to receive ceftazidime for a lung infection. References indicate that the safe dose of ceftazidime is 50 mg/kg every 8 hours. What is the recommended single dose?

20. A patient is to receive 20 units of Pitocin® in 500 mL of lactated Ringer's. The IV is to run at a rate of 3 units/hour. How many milliliters per hour should the infusion pump be set to?

**21.** A physician writes an order for 40 g of magnesium sulfate to be added to a liter of D5W. The patient is to receive 3.5 g of magnesium sulfate per hour. How many milliliters per hour should be administered?

**22.** The label on fluconazole oral suspension indicates that 24 mL of water should be added to the dry powder to make 35 mL of a solution containing 10 mg/mL.

(a) What is the volume of the dry powder?

(b) How many grams of fluconazole are contained in a full bottle?

(c) How many milliliters of the suspension should a 48-lb child receive if the package insert indicates the dose is 3 mg/kg?

**23.** Dopamine is infusing at 15 mL/hour. The bag contains 400 mg in 0.25 liter of D5W.

(a) How many grams of dopamine is the patient receiving per hour?

(b) How many micrograms per kilogram per minute is the patient receiving if she weighs 163 lb?

(c) For how many minutes will this IV run before the bag is empty?

**24.** Ipratropium bromide is available in a 0.02% concentration. How many milligrams are contained in a 2.5-mL vial of ipratropium bromide?

**25.** An 8.2-lb baby is to receive 0.05 mg/kg of Adenocard®. The drug is supplied as a 6-mg/2-mL solution.

  (a) What volume will deliver the required dose?

  (b) What volume will provide the desired dose if the drug has been diluted to 0.003 g/10 mL?

*You should be well prepared to tackle the PI challenge & Posttests!*

Now, I want you to take the ultimate challenge. The following questions were developed directly from pharmaceutical product package inserts (PIs). These questions will give you an opportunity to see how well you can interpret the information provided by pharmaceutical manufacturers. I'm confident that you are well prepared and can handle these real-world calculation problems.

*GOOD LUCK with the PI Challenge!!!*

**26.** After the first 24 hours, the maintenance infusion rate of amiodarone hydrochloride injection is 0.5 mg/minute. Express this rate as grams per day.

**27.** Out of a total of 1936 patients in controlled and uncontrolled clinical trials, 14% received 300 mg of an investigational drug daily for at least 1 week. How many patients received the 300-mg/day dose?

**28.** The package insert for calcium gluconate injection 10% states that infants should not receive more than 200 mg of calcium gluconate. How many milliliters would this be?

**29.** The recommended adult dose of benzonatate for symptomatic relief of cough is one 100-mg or 200-mg capsule t.i.d. as required. If necessary, up to 600 mg daily may be given. What is the maximum number of 100-mg capsules that should be dispensed for 1 week of therapy?

**30.** In patients with normal renal function, peak serum concentrations of gentamicin (mcg/mL) are usually up to four times the single IM dose (mg/kg); for example, a 1-mg/kg injection in adults may be expected to result in a peak serum concentration of up to 4 mcg/mL. What estimated peak serum concentration would result from a 1.7-mg/kg dose for a life-threatening infection?

**31.** How many gentamicin 80-mg/2-mL vials are required daily to provide a 176-lb patient with a 1-mg/kg dose q.8 hours?

**32.** Ipratropium bromide inhalation solution 0.02% is available in 2.5-mL vials. How many milligrams of ipratropium bromide are in each vial?

**33.** Exceeding the recommended dose of phenazopyridine hydrochloride in patients with good renal function or administering the usual dose to patients with impaired renal function (commonly seen in elderly patients) may lead to increased serum levels and toxic reactions. Methemoglobinemia generally follows a massive, acute overdose. Methylene blue, 1 to 2 mg/kg body weight intravenously, or ascorbic acid, 100 to 200 mg given orally, should cause prompt reduction of methemoglobinemia. What is the maximum dose of methylene blue recommended for an unconscious 198-lb patient?

**34.** Transdermal scopolamine patches contain 1.5 mg of scopolamine and are programmed to deliver in vivo approximately 1 mg of scopolamine over 3 days. How many micrograms of scopolamine would a patient receive daily from a patch?

**35.** Succinylcholine chloride injection is available in a 10-mL multidose vial containing 20 mg/mL. The average dose required to produce neuromuscular blockade and to facilitate tracheal intubation is 0.6 mg/kg intravenously. How many milliliters would be administered to a 154-lb patient?

36. The PI for a drug states to "store at 2 to 8°C." Convert this "range" to degrees Fahrenheit; should you store this drug in the freezer, in the refrigerator, or at room temperature?

37. A loading infusion containing 20 mg/mL of procainamide hydrochloride (1 g diluted to 50 mL with 5% dextrose injection USP) may be administered at a constant rate of 1 mL/minute for 25 to 30 minutes. How many milligrams of procainamide hydrochloride would a patient receive in 25 minutes?

38. Plasma levels of procainamide hydrochloride above 10 mcg/mL are increasingly associated with toxic findings. Express this plasma level in grams per liter.

39. The recommended starting dose of levothyroxine sodium in newborn infants is 10 mcg/kg/day. How many milligrams would be given to a 6.6-lb infant?

40. Angioedema of the face, lips, tongue, glottis, and/or larynx has been reported in patients treated with angiotensin-converting enzyme inhibitors. Angioedema associated with laryngeal edema may be fatal. Where there is involvement of the tongue, glottis, or larynx likely to cause airway obstruction, appropriate therapy, e.g., subcutaneous epinephrine solution 1:1000 (0.3 to 0.5 mL), should be promptly provided. How many milligrams of epinephrine would a patient receive from the highest dose?

41. In a zoledronic acid clinical study, patients were given a loading dose of vitamin D (50,000 to 125,000 IU orally or IM) and were then started on 1000 to 1500 mg of elemental calcium plus 800 to 1200 IU of vitamin D supplementation per day for at least 14 days prior to the infusion of the study drug. What is the minimum amount of vitamin D a patient could have received in this study?

**42.** Patients with ulcerative proctitis were given one mesalamine 500-mg rectal suppository every 8 hours for 6 days during pharmacokinetic elimination studies.

(a) How many grams of mesalamine did each patient receive?

(b) Approximately 12% of the 6-day dose was eliminated in the urine as unchanged 5-ASA. How many milligrams of 5-ASA were eliminated unchanged in the urine?

**43.** Hyoscyamine sulfate is supplied as 0.125-mg tablets. Adults can receive one to two tablets every 4 hours or as needed, not to exceed 12 tablets in 24 hours. How many micrograms of hyoscyamine sulfate would a patient receive if he took half of the maximum daily dose?

**44.** According to the PI, the maintenance infusion rate of 0.75 mg/minute of clindamycin will maintain a serum level of about 4 mcg/mL. How many grams of clindamycin would a patient receive in a day to maintain the 4-mcg/mL serum level?

**45.** A 5-lb neonate is to receive 15 mg/kg/day of an antibiotic in 4 equal doses. How much will the baby receive in a single dose?

**46.** The label on an antibiotic states: "store dry powder below 86°F." Express this temperature in degrees centigrade. Should this powder be stored in a refrigerator, in a freezer, or at room temperature?

**47.** In three double-blind controlled studies conducted in the United States, azithromycin (12 mg/kg once daily for 5 days) was compared to penicillin V (250 mg three times a day for 10 days) in the treatment of pharyngitis. Azithromycin had a bacteriologic eradication rate of 323 out of 340 patients. Penicillin V had a bacteriologic eradication rate of 242 out of 332 patients. Express these bacteriologic eradication rates as percentages and determine which product was more effective.

**48.** Folbic™ tablets are a medical food for the dietary management of hyper-homocysteinemia. Each tablet contains the following active ingredients: folacin 2.5 mg, pyridoxine hydrochloride 25 mg, and cyanocobalamin 2 mg. How many total grams of active ingredients would a patient receive from one tablet daily for 30 days?

**49.** Labetalol hydrochloride injection 5 mg/mL is supplied in 20-mL multidose vials. For slow continuous infusion, the contents of two 20-mL vials are added to 260 mL of a commonly used intravenous fluid.

(a) What is the resultant concentration of labetalol hydrochloride in this solution in milligrams per milliliter?

(b) The diluted solution is to be administered at a rate to deliver 2 mg/minute. How many milliliters of the diluted solution will the patient receive in 30 minutes?

**50.** Octreotide acetate injection is available as sterile 5-mL multidose vials in two strengths containing 200 and 1000 mcg/mL of octreotide.

(a) How many milligrams of octreotide are contained in the lowest concentration vial?

(b) The multidose vials also contain 5 mg/mL of phenol USP. Express the concentration of phenol USP as a percent strength.

**51.** In a clinical drug study, 12% of patients (n = 87) developed arrhythmias after 7 days on an experimental medication. Based on this information, how many patients participated in the study? (Hint: "n = 87" means that 87 patients developed arrhythmias.)

**52.** Hydrocortisone acetate rectal suppositories each contain hydrocortisone acetate USP 25 mg in a specially blended hydrogenated vegetable oil base. In normal subjects, about 26% of hydrocortisone acetate is absorbed when the suppository is applied to the rectum. How many milligrams would be absorbed if a patient inserts one suppository into the rectum twice daily for 2 weeks?

**53.** Magnesium sulfate injection USP (50%) for IV and IM use is a sterile concentrated solution of magnesium sulfate. How many milligrams of magnesium sulfate is in a milliliter of this solution?

**54.** Isoproterenol hydrochloride injection USP is available in a 1:5000 strength. How much of this injection should be given to deliver a 0.2-mg subcutaneous initial dose?

**55.** Approximately 5% of a subcutaneous dose of vasopressin is excreted in the urine unchanged after 4 hours. How much vasopressin would a normal patient excrete in the urine 4 hours after a 0.5-mL subcutaneous dose if there are 5 units of vasopressin in 0.25 mL of the injection?

**56.** According to the PI warnings section, serious rash associated with hospitalization and discontinuation of lamotrigine occurred in 11 of 3348 adult patients who received lamotrigine in premarketing clinical trials of this epilepsy drug. Express this incidence of serious rash as a percentage.

**57.** Somnolence as an adverse reaction was recorded during controlled hypertension studies comparing doxazosin mesylate to a placebo. Doxazosin had a 5% incidence among the 339 patients receiving the drug. There was a 1% incidence among the 336 patients receiving the placebo. Approximately how many more patients experienced somnolence in the doxazosin group compared to the placebo group?

**58.** Daily doses of 200 mg of prednisolone for a week followed by 80 mg every other day for 1 month have been shown to be effective in the treatment of acute exacerbations of multiple sclerosis.

(a) How many grams of prednisolone would a patient following this protocol receive?

(b) If 4 mg of methylprednisolone is equivalent to 5 mg of prednisolone, how many grams of methylprednisolone would a multiple sclerosis patient receive during the first week of therapy?

**59.** The recommended dose of pregabalin for fibromyalgia is 300 to 450 mg/day. Dosing should begin at 75 mg two times a day (150 mg/day), and it may be increased to 150 mg two times a day (300 mg/day) after 1 week based on efficacy and tolerability. How many 75-mg pregabalin capsules will need to be dispensed for 14 days if a patient follows this titration protocol?

**60.** Montelukast sodium 4-mg oral granules can be dissolved in 1 teaspoonful (5 mL) of cold or room-temperature baby formula or breast milk. How many micrograms of montelukast sodium will be in a drop of this mixture if a dropper delivers 12 drops per milliliter?

**61.** According to the PI, each vial of drotrecogin alfa (activated) should be reconstituted with sterile water for injection USP. The 5-mg vials must be reconstituted with 2.5 mL; the 20-mg vials should be reconstituted with 10 mL. Sterile water for injection USP should be slowly added to the vial, and the vial should not be inverted or shaken. Each vial is swirled until the powder is completely dissolved. The resulting drotrecogin alfa concentration of the solution is 2 mg/mL. What is the dry powder volume represented by the drug in the 20-mg vial?

**62.** The neonatal dosage regimen of vancomycin is a 15-mg/kg initial dose followed by 10 mg/kg every 12 hours.

(a) What is the initial dose for an infant weighing 7 lb 3 oz?

(b) What is the subsequent dose for this infant?

(c) If the doses are obtained from a 500-mg vial of vancomycin that has been reconstituted to a concentration of 50 mg/mL, what volume will give the required initial dose?

(d) What volume will this patient receive daily for the subsequent doses?

**63.** An intravenous infusion of magnesium sulfate can be prepared by adding 4 g of magnesium sulfate from a concentrated solution to 250 mL of 5% dextrose. The maximum infusion rate should not exceed 3 mL/minute. How many milligrams of magnesium sulfate will a patient receive per hour based on the maximum infusion rate?

NOTE: The change in volume is negligible when adding the concentrated solution.

64. Calfactant intratracheal suspension should only be administered intratracheally through an endotracheal tube. The dose is 3 mL/kg of birth weight. Each milliliter of this suspension contains 35 mg of total phospholipids. This suspension is supplied in sterile 3- and 6-mL vials. How many milligrams of phospholipids would a 6.6-lb newborn receive?

65. In dietary administration studies in which mice and rats were treated with propranolol for up to 18 months at doses of up to 150 mg/kg/day, there was no evidence of drug-related tumorigenesis. How many grams of propranolol would a 185-g rodent receive in 1 year, assuming maximum daily doses?

66. Triamcinolone acetonide cream USP 0.025% is available in 15- and 80-g tubes. How many pounds of triamcinolone acetonide would be required to manufacture 10,000 of the larger tubes?

67. Patients receiving niacin extended-release tablets are dosed with an initial titration schedule to reduce the incidence and severity of side effects which may occur during early therapy. The recommended dose escalation is 500 mg at bedtime for weeks 1 through 4 and 1000 mg at bedtime for weeks 5 through 8. How many 500-mg tablets would be dispensed for this 2-month titration?

68. Absorption of tamsulosin hydrochloride is essentially complete (90%) following oral administration under fasting conditions. Approximately how much tamsulosin will be absorbed in 30 days if a patient takes the recommended dose of 0.4 mg once daily?

**69.** In overdosage studies, doses of 2.5 mg of octreotide acetate injection subcutaneously have caused hypoglycemia, flushing, dizziness, and nausea. The recommended starting dose for acromegaly is 50 mcg three times a day. How many times the recommended daily dose was the dose used in the overdosage studies?

**70.** Magnesium sulfate injection USP contains 4.06 mEq of magnesium sulfate per milliliter.

   (a) How many milligrams of magnesium sulfate is in a 10-mL vial of this injection? (MW = 246, valence = 2)

   (b) What is the percent strength of the magnesium sulfate injection?

**71.** The recommended initial intravenous infusion dose of isoproterenol hydrochloride injection 1:5000 for Adams-Stokes attacks is 5 mcg/minute. How many milliliters of a diluted 1:5000 injection should be administered to deliver the recommended dose?

   NOTE: To prepare this infusion, dilute 10 mL (2 mg) of isoproterenol hydrochloride injection in 5% dextrose injection USP to make a final volume of 500 mL.

**72.** In vivo studies in healthy volunteers confirm that ranolazine is primarily metabolized by CYP3A. Plasma levels of ranolazine with 1000-mg b.i.d. doses are increased 3.2-fold by the potent CYP3A inhibitor ketoconazole coadministered at a dose of 200 mg b.i.d. Express this increase in plasma levels as a percentage.

73. For diuresis and for control of hypertension in infants and children, the usual pediatric dosage of hydrochlorothiazide is 0.5 to 1 mg/lb/day in a single dose or two divided doses, not to exceed 100 mg/day in children 2 to 12 years of age. How much would a 23-kg 6-year-old child receive in a single dose if the physician prescribed the maximum recommended daily dose given b.i.d.?

74. Albuterol sulfate inhalation solution is available in a 2.5-mg/0.5-mL strength.

   (a) Express this concentration as a percent strength.

   (b) Express this concentration as a ratio strength.

75. The precautions section of the ketoconazole cream PI cites the incidence of hepatitis caused by use of this cream to be 1:10,000. Based on this information, how many potential cases of hepatitis could occur if 3,870,000 patients worldwide use ketoconazole cream?

76. In infants (up to 2 years of age), a 4.2% sodium bicarbonate injection is recommended for intravenous administration at a dose not to exceed 8 mEq/kg/day. What is the maximum amount in milliliters that a 10-kg infant can receive in a day? (MW = 84, valence = 1)

77. Each milliliter of norepinephrine bitartrate injection contains the equivalent of 1 mg of norepinephrine base and approximately 2 mg of sodium metabisulfite as an antioxidant. What is the combined percent strength of norepinephrine and sodium metabisulfite in this injection?

**78.** Cefazolin for injection USP is available in vials containing cefazolin sodium equivalent to 500 mg or 1 g of cefazolin. The 1-g vial must be reconstituted with 2.5 mL of sterile water for injection. The approximate available volume after reconstitution is 3 mL.

(a) What is the dry powder volume of cefazolin?

(b) How many milligrams of cefazolin are in 1 mL of the reconstituted vial?

**79.** Following oral administration of 200 mg of a radioactive dose of bupropion in humans, 87% and 10% of the radioactive dose were recovered in the urine and the feces, respectively. Approximately how many grams of bupropion were recovered in the feces?

**80.** To prepare diltiazem hydrochloride injection for continuous intravenous infusion, the appropriate quantity of the injection is aseptically transferred to the desired volume of normal saline. If 250 mg (50 mL) of diltiazem hydrochloride injection is added to 500 mL of diluent, what is the approximate final concentration in milligrams per milliliter?

**81.** The clinical studies data in the PI for raloxifene hydrochloride compare the effects of raloxifene and a placebo on the risk of vertebral fractures. One of the raloxifene studies evaluated the number of new vertebral fractures. In this study, there were 1401 patients receiving raloxifene and 1457 receiving a placebo. How many more patients in the placebo group had fractures compared to the raloxifene group if there was a 4.3% incidence of fracture in patients receiving a placebo compared to 1.9% in patients receiving raloxifene?

82. The PI for hydrocortisone states that hydrocortisone USP is a white, odorless powder with a melting point of about 215°C. Express this melting point as degrees Fahrenheit.

83. Immune globulin intravenous (human) 10% is infused at an initial rate of 0.5 mL/kg/hr. Express this rate as milligrams per kilogram per minute.

84. Phenytoin sodium injection is indicated for the control of status epilepticus of the grand mal type and for prevention and treatment of seizures occurring during neurosurgery. Phenytoin injection is available in 5-mL single-use vials, each containing 250 mg of phenytoin sodium. The recommended loading dose for adults with status epilepticus is 10 to 15 mg/kg. The infusion rate should not exceed 50 mg/minute. The maximum adult dose is given to a 191-lb patient and is diluted in 250 mL of normal saline (NS).

    (a) What is the total dose for this patient?

    (b) What is the shortest time in which this dose can be infused?

    (c) How many vials of phenytoin sodium will be needed to provide the total dose?

    (d) What is the approximate volume of the diluted solution?

    (e) How many milliliters per minute will this patient receive?

    (f) How many micrograms per minute of phenytoin sodium will this patient receive?

**85.** The pediatric dose of adenosine for patients with a body weight < 50 kg is 0.05 to 0.1 mg/kg as a rapid IV bolus. This product is supplied in 2-mL vials containing 6 mg of adenosine.

    (a) What is the lowest recommended dose for a child weighing 19 lb 4 oz?

    (b) What volume would deliver the lowest recommended dose?

**86.** Albuterol sulfate inhalation solution 0.5% is in concentrated form. Instructions state to dilute 0.5 mL of the solution to 3 mL with sterile normal saline (NS) solution prior to administration.

    (a) What is the percent strength of the final solution?

    (b) What would be the percent strength of the solution if you accidentally added 0.5 mL of albuterol solution to 3 mL of NS?

**87.** Clarithromycin for oral suspension requires water to be added when reconstituting. The 100-mL bottle of 250-mg/5-mL concentration requires 55 mL of water to be added.

    (a) What is the dry powder volume of the clarithromycin?

    (b) How many grams of clarithromycin are in the bottle?

    (c) What would be the concentration of clarithromycin in milligrams per teaspoon if you accidentally added 85 mL of water?

**88.** In postmarketing experience, injection site cellulitislike reactions were reported rarely with the pneumococcal vaccine. Between 1989 and 2002, when approximately 43 million doses were distributed, the annual reporting rate was less than 2/100,000 doses. These cellulitislike reactions occurred with initial and repeat vaccination at a median onset time of 2 days after vaccine administration.

(a) Express the reporting rate as a percentage.

(b) Estimate the total number of cellulitislike reactions.

**89.** The following are instructions for the administration of mupirocin calcium ointment 2%:

Approximately one-half of the ointment from the single-use tube should be applied into one nostril and the other half into the other nostril. The ointment should be applied twice daily (morning and evening) for 5 days. The single-use 1-g tube will deliver a total of approximately 0.5 gram of ointment (approximately 0.25 gram/nostril).

(a) What is the ratio strength of the mupirocin calcium ointment?

(b) What is the ratio strength of mupirocin calcium in one nostril?

**90.** Fluconazole injection may be administered by intravenous infusion and can be administered at a maximum rate of approximately 200 mg/hour, given as a continuous infusion. This antifungal agent is available as fluconazole in sodium chloride diluent 400 mg/200 mL.

(a) How many milliliters per minute would be required to provide the maximum recommended rate of infusion?

(b) How many drops per minute will be required to administer that dose if the IV set delivers 15 gtt/mL?

**91.** The recommended daily dosage of cephalexin for pediatric patients in the treatment of otitis media is 75 to 100 mg/kg/day in 4 divided doses.

    (a) How many grams of cephalexin would a 44-lb patient receive daily if he received the maximum recommended dose?

    (b) How many milligrams per dose would this 44-lb patient receive?

    (c) How many milliliters of a 250-mg/tsp cephalexin suspension would this patient receive daily?

**92.** Gatifloxacin ophthalmic solution contains gatifloxacin 0.3% as the active ingredient and benzalkonium chloride 0.005% as a preservative.

    (a) What is the gatifloxacin concentration in milligrams per milliliter?

    (b) Express the preservative concentration as a ratio strength.

**93.** If only the earliest manifestations of diabetic gastric stasis are present, oral administration of metoclopramide may be initiated. However, if severe symptoms are present, therapy should begin with metoclopramide injection (IM or IV). Doses of 10 mg may be administered slowly by the intravenous route over a 1- to 2-minute period. Administration of metoclopramide injection USP for up to 10 days may be required before symptoms subside, at which time oral administration of metoclopramide may be instituted. Metoclopramide is available in 2-mL flip-top glass vials containing 5 mg/mL.

    (a) How many vials would be required to provide 1 dose a day for 1 week?

    (b) What is the percent strength of metoclopramide?

**94.** Ropivacaine hydrochloride injection 0.75% is available in 20-mL ampules. The dose of this local anesthetic varies with the anesthetic procedure, the area to be anesthetized, the vascularity of the tissue, and other factors. The dose range for a brachial plexus block is 75 to 300 mg.

(a) How many grams of ropivacaine hydrochloride are contained in an ampule?

(b) How many milliliters would be required to administer the maximum dose?

**95.** Reconstituted caspofungin acetate for injection has a concentration of 7.2 mg/mL. Ten milliliters of this reconstituted solution is aseptically transferred to an IV bag containing 250 mL of 0.9% sodium chloride injection. What is the final concentration of caspofungin in milligrams per milliliter?

**96.** Somnolence was the most common treatment-emergent adverse event associated with the use of ziprasidone in 4- and 6-week trials for schizophrenia. If 14% of the 702 patients reported experiencing somnolence, how many patients did not report this adverse event?

**97.** Propofol injectable emulsion is a sterile, nonpyrogenic emulsion containing 10 mg/mL of propofol suitable for intravenous administration. The dosing guidelines indicate that a dose of 100 to 200 mcg/kg/minute can be used for the maintenance of general anesthesia in healthy adults less than 55 years of age.

(a) Express this dosing range in milligrams per kilogram per hour.

(b) How many milliliters would provide the minimum dose for 1 hour for a 60-kg patient?

**98.** The recommended IV dosage of ondansetron for adults for prevention of chemotherapy-induced nausea and vomiting is three 0.15-mg/kg doses. The first dose is infused over 15 minutes, beginning 30 minutes before the start of emetogenic chemotherapy. Subsequent doses are administered 4 and 8 hours after the first dose of ondansetron.

(a) How many 4-mg/2-mL single-dose vials will be needed to administer the first dose for a 72-kg patient?

(b) How many milliliters must be infused to provide the entire dosage regimen?

**99.** The usual pediatric dose of amoxicillin suspension for severe genitourinary tract infections is 40 mg/kg/day in divided doses every 8 hours.

(a) How many milligrams would a 53-lb patient receive in each dose?

(b) How many milliliters should this patient receive to provide the appropriate dose if the pharmacy dispenses a 100-mL bottle of amoxicillin 400 mg/tsp?

(c) Will the dispensed bottle provide 10 days of therapy?

**100.** Last, but not least...

***you must now save your own life!!!***

You are shipwrecked on an isolated South Pacific island with little to no possibility of ever being rescued. You have contracted an incredibly painful and horribly disfiguring tropical disease that will be fatal if left untreated.

*Believe it or not, this is your lucky day!*

A bottle of a rare antibiotic has washed up on the beach and just happens to be "in date" and the only drug known to treat your ailment. The label says to reconstitute the antibiotic with 129 mL of water to make 200 mL of a solution containing 350 mg of antibiotic per teaspoonful. In your excitement, you accidentally use 159 mL of water to reconstitute the antibiotic. Normally, this would not be a disastrous error, but this is an unusual antibiotic, in that the dose must be accurate. A 5% error in dosing can render the drug ineffective if dosed too low, and too-high doses can lead to fatal renal and hepatic failure as well as terrible seizures. The pressure is on **you** due to your compounding error.

(a) You must now determine how many milliliters of the incorrectly compounded antibiotic will be required in each dose to deliver 350 mg q.i.d. × 10 days.

*Good Luck!!!*

Bonus:

(b) Will you have enough antibiotic to complete the full course of therapy?

# Appendix

## ISMP List of Error-Prone Abbreviations, Symbols, and Dose Designations[a]

| Abbreviations | Intended Meaning | Misinterpretation | Correction |
|---|---|---|---|
| μg | Microgram | Mistaken as "mg" | Use "mcg" |
| AD, AS, AU | Right ear, left ear, each ear | Mistaken as OD, OS, OU (right eye, left eye, each eye) | Use "right ear," "left ear," or "each ear" |
| OD, OS, OU | Right eye, left eye, each eye | Mistaken as AD, AS, AU (right ear, left ear, each ear) | Use "right eye," "left eye," or "each eye" |
| BT | Bedtime | Mistaken as "BID" (twice daily) | Use "bedtime" |
| cc | Cubic centimeters | Mistaken as "u" (units) | Use "mL" |
| D/C | Discharge or discontinue | Premature discontinuation of medications if D/C (intended to mean "discharge") has been misinterpreted as "discontinued" when followed by a list of discharge medications | Use "discharge" and "discontinue" |
| IJ | Injection | Mistaken as "IV" or "intrajugular" | Use "injection" |
| IN | Intranasal | Mistaken as "IM" or "IV" | Use "intranasal" or "NAS" |
| HS | Half-strength | Mistaken as bedtime | Use "half-strength" or "bedtime" |
| hs | At bedtime, hours of sleep | Mistaken as half-strength | |
| IU[b] | International unit | Mistaken as IV (intravenous) or 10 (ten) | Use "units" |
| o.d. or OD | Once daily | Mistaken as "right eye" (OD-oculus dexter), leading to oral liquid medications administered in the eye | Use "daily" |
| OJ | Orange juice | Mistaken as OD or OS (right or left eye); drugs meant to be diluted in orange juice may be given in the eye | Use "orange juice" |
| Per os | By mouth, orally | The "os" can be mistaken as "left eye" (OS-oculus sinister) | Use "PO," "by mouth," or "orally" |
| q.d. or QD[b] | Every day | Mistaken as q.i.d., especially if the period after the "q" or the tail of the "q" is misunderstood as an "i" | Use "daily" |
| qhs | Nightly at bedtime | Mistaken as "qhr" or every hour | Use "nightly" |
| qn | Nightly or at bedtime | Mistaken as "qh" (every hour) | Use "nightly" or "at bedtime" |
| q.o.d. or QOD[b] | Every other day | Mistaken as "q.d." (daily) or "q.i.d. (four times daily) if the "o" is poorly written | Use "every other day" |
| q1d | Daily | Mistaken as q.i.d. (four times daily) | Use "daily" |
| q6PM, etc. | Every evening at 6 PM | Mistaken as every 6 hours | Use "6 PM nightly" or "6 PM daily" |
| SC, SQ, sub q | Subcutaneous | SC mistaken as SL (sublingual); SQ mistaken as "5 every;" the "q" in "sub q" has been mistaken as "every" (e.g., a heparin dose ordered "sub q 2 hours before surgery" misunderstood as every 2 hours before surgery) | Use "subcut" or "subcutaneously" |
| ss | Sliding scale (insulin) or ½ (apothecary) | Mistaken as "55" | Spell out "sliding scale;" use "one-half" or "½" |
| SSRI | Sliding scale regular insulin | Mistaken as selective-serotonin reuptake inhibitor | Spell out "sliding scale (insulin)" |
| SSI | Sliding scale insulin | Mistaken as Strong Solution of Iodine (Lugol's) | |
| 1/d | One daily | Mistaken as "tid" | Use "1 daily" |
| TIW or tiw | 3 times a week | Mistaken as "3 times a day" or "twice in a week" | Use "3 times weekly" |
| U or u[b] | Unit | Mistaken as the number 0 or 4, causing a 10-fold overdose or greater (e.g., 4U seen as "40" or 4u seen as "44"); mistaken as "cc" so dose given in volume instead of units (e.g., 4u seen as 4cc) | Use "unit" |

| Dose Designations and Other Information | Intended Meaning | Misinterpretation | Correction |
|---|---|---|---|
| Trailing zero after decimal point (e.g., 1.0 mg)[b] | 1 mg | Mistaken as 10 mg if the decimal point is not seen | Do not use trailing zeros for doses expressed in whole numbers |
| No leading zero before a decimal dose (e.g., .5 mg)[b] | 0.5 mg | Mistaken as 5 mg if the decimal point is not seen | Use zero before a decimal point when the dose is less than a whole unit |

*continues on next page*

| Dose Designations and Other Information | Intended Meaning | Misinterpretation | Correction |
|---|---|---|---|
| Drug name and dose run together (especially problematic for drug names that end in "L" such as Inderal40 mg; Tegretol300 mg) | Inderal 40 mg<br><br>Tegretol 300 mg | Mistaken as Inderal 140 mg<br><br>Mistaken as Tegretol 1300 mg | Place adequate space between the drug name, dose, and unit of measure |
| Numerical dose and unit of measure run together (e.g., 10mg, 100mL) | 10 mg<br><br>100 mL | The "m" is sometimes mistaken as a zero or two zeros, risking a 10- to 100-fold overdose | Place adequate space between the dose and unit of measure |
| Abbreviations such as mg. or mL. with a period following the abbreviation | mg<br><br>mL | The period is unnecessary and could be mistaken as the number 1 if written poorly | Use mg, mL, etc. without a terminal period |
| Large doses without properly placed commas (e.g., 100000 units; 1000000 units) | 100,000 units<br><br>1,000,000 units | 100000 has been mistaken as 10,000 or 1,000,000; 1000000 has been mistaken as 100,000 | Use commas for dosing units at or above 1,000, or use words such as 100 "thousand" or 1 "million" to improve readability |

| Drug Name Abbreviations | Intended Meaning | Misinterpretation | Correction |
|---|---|---|---|
| ARA A | vidarabine | Mistaken as cytarabine (ARA C) | Use complete drug name |
| AZT | zidovudine (Retrovir) | Mistaken as azathioprine or aztreonam | Use complete drug name |
| CPZ | Compazine (prochlorperazine) | Mistaken as chlorpromazine | Use complete drug name |
| DPT | Demerol-Phenergan-Thorazine | Mistaken as diphtheria-pertussis-tetanus (vaccine) | Use complete drug name |
| DTO | Diluted tincture of opium, or deodorized tincture of opium (Paregoric) | Mistaken as tincture of opium | Use complete drug name |
| HCl | hydrochloric acid or hydrochloride | Mistaken as potassium chloride (The "H" is misinterpreted as "K") | Use complete drug name unless expressed as a salt of a drug |
| HCT | hydrocortisone | Mistaken as hydrochlorothiazide | Use complete drug name |
| HCTZ | hydrochlorothiazide | Mistaken as hydrocortisone (seen as HCT250 mg) | Use complete drug name |
| MgSO4 [b] | magnesium sulfate | Mistaken as morphine sulfate | Use complete drug name |
| MS, MSO4 [b] | morphine sulfate | Mistaken as magnesium sulfate | Use complete drug name |
| MTX | methotrexate | Mistaken as mitoxantrone | Use complete drug name |
| PCA | procainamide | Mistaken as Patient Controlled Analgesia | Use complete drug name |
| PTU | propylthiouracil | Mistaken as mercaptopurine | Use complete drug name |
| T3 | Tylenol with codeine No. 3 | Mistaken as liothyronine | Use complete drug name |
| TAC | triamcinolone | Mistaken as tetracaine, Adrenalin, cocaine | Use complete drug name |
| TNK | TNKase | Mistaken as "TPA" | Use complete drug name |
| ZnSO4 | zinc sulfate | Mistaken as morphine sulfate | Use complete drug name |

| Stemmed Drug Names | Intended Meaning | Misinterpretation | Correction |
|---|---|---|---|
| "Nitro" drip | nitroglycerin infusion | Mistaken as sodium nitroprusside infusion | Use complete drug name |
| "Norflox" | norfloxacin | Mistaken as Norflex | Use complete drug name |
| "IV Vanc" | intravenous vancomycin | Mistaken as Invanz | Use complete drug name |

| Symbols | Intended Meaning | Misinterpretation | Correction |
|---|---|---|---|
| ʒ | Dram | Symbol for dram mistaken as "3" | Use the metric system |
| ♏ | Minim | Symbol for minim mistaken as "mL" | |
| x3d | For three days | Mistaken as "3 doses" | Use "for three days" |
| > and < | Greater than and less than | Mistaken as opposite of intended; mistakenly use incorrect symbol; "< 10" mistaken as "40" | Use "greater than" or "less than" |
| / (slash mark) | Separates two doses or indicates "per" | Mistaken as the number 1 (e.g., "25 units/10 units" misread as "25 units and 110 units) | Use "per" rather than a slash mark to separate doses |
| @ | At | Mistaken as "2" | Use "at" |
| & | And | Mistaken as "2" | Use "and" |
| + | Plus or and | Mistaken as "4" | Use "and" |
| ° | Hour | Mistaken as a zero (e.g., q2° seen as q 20) | Use "hr," "h," or "hour" |

[a] Originally published in ISMP Medication Safety Alert!® 2003; 8: 3–4. ©Institute for Safe Medication Practices. All rights reserved. Reprinted with permission.

[b] Abbreviation also on the Joint Commission's "minimum list" of dangerous abbreviations, acronyms, and symbols that must be included on an organization's "Do Not Use" list, effective January 1, 2004. An updated list of frequently asked questions about this requirement can be found at www.jointcommission.org.

# Posttest I: Mega Math Marathon

It has been a pleasure helping you overcome the barriers associated with learning pharmaceutical calculations. If you have mastered the material in this textbook, you will be able to answer the majority of questions you will encounter in pharmacy practice.

This penultimate section is designed to give you a chance to solve real-world problems and evaluate how knowledgeable you have become about pharmacy math. Please work the following problems slowly and carefully. Do not work these questions until you have mastered _all_ the objectives in this textbook. You have been prepared for each of these 101 questions (events), but in some cases, you will have to search a little to find the information you need (such as molecular weights and labeling information). Read every question carefully. I will constantly attempt to trick you into making a careless error. When you finish this posttest, add up all your correct "event" answers and score yourself as follows:

**GOLD MEDAL** (90–101): _You are awesome!_

**SILVER MEDAL** (80–89): _You should be very proud of yourself!_

**BRONZE MEDAL** (70–79): _You are doing well, but you could do better!_

If you score below 70, you need to practice, practice, practice. Then return to this chapter and try again. Hopefully, you will be in contention for a medal next time.

Just remember, **_you are a winner_** for studying and for trying to improve your skills.

_I WISH YOU THE BEST OF LUCK IN YOUR PHARMACY CAREER._

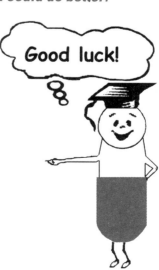

Good luck!

# Now, Let The Marathon Begin!

**For events 1–3:**

| Canine Diarrhea Capsules | |
| --- | --- |
| **R**℞ *(For 100 capsules)* | |
| Neomycin sulfate | 1.44 g |
| Sulfaguanidine | 14.8 g |
| Sulfadiazine | 920 mg |
| Sulfamerazine | 920 mg |
| Sulfathiazole | 920 mg |
| Kaolin | 30 g |
| Pectin | 1 g |

Courtesy of *International Journal of Pharmaceutical Compounding*

1. How many milligrams of neomycin sulfate are contained in one capsule?

2. What is the percent strength of neomycin sulfate in this formula?

3. How many milligrams of kaolin would be required to prepare 30 capsules?

**For events 4 & 5:**

**Flovent® 110 mcg**
**(fluticasone propionate, 110 mcg) Inhalation Aerosol**
FOR ORAL INHALATION ONLY
Canister is to be used with Flovent® Inhalation Aerosol actuator only.

Attention: **Dispense with enclosed "Patient's Instructions for Use"**

**See package outsert for full prescribing information.**
Rx only

Net Wt. 13 g
120 Metered Actuations

4. How many milligrams of fluticasone propionate are in a canister?

5. What is the percent strength of fluticasone propionate in this canister?

**For events 6 & 7:**

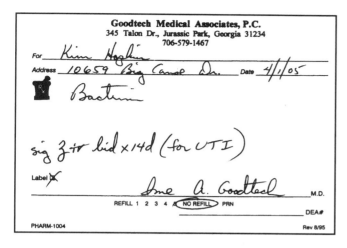

**6.** How many milliliters of Bactrim® suspension would you dispense?

**7.** Bactrim suspension contains 200 mg of sulfamethoxazole and 40 mg of trimethoprim per 5 mL. How many total grams of the drugs will Kim receive daily?

**For events 8 & 9:**

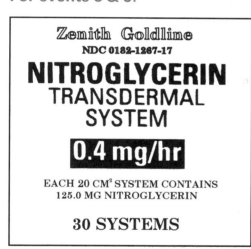

**8.** How many micrograms of nitroglycerin will a patient receive in 12 hours?

**9.** How many grams of nitroglycerin are in all of the systems in this box?

**For events 10–12:**

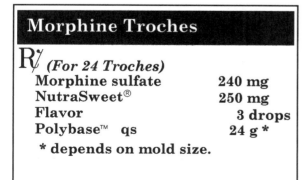

Courtesy of *International Journal of Pharmaceutical Compounding*

**10.** How many milligrams of morphine are in each troche?

**11.** What is the mg% of morphine sulfate in this formulation?

**12.** How many grams of NutraSweet® are required to prepare 100 troches?

**For events 13–15:**

| | |
|---|---|
| USUAL DOSAGE: Apply to the affected area as a thin film from two to four times daily depending on the severity of the condition. Store at controlled room temperature 15°- 30°C (59°-86°F). Avoid excessive heat above °C (104°F)<br><br>See package insert for full prescribing information.<br>**E. FOUGERA & CO.**<br>a division of Altana Inc. MELVILLE, NEW YORK 11747b<br>**NDC** 0168-0139-30<br>**fougera** ®<br>**FLUOCINONIDE**<br>**CREAM USP, 0.05%** | To Open: To puncture the seal, reverse the cap and place the puncture-top onto the tube. Push down firmly until seal is open. To close, screw the cap back onto the tube.<br>**CAUTION:** Federal law prohibits dispensing without prescription.<br>WARNING: Keep out of reach of children.<br>**FOR EXTERNAL USE ONLY. NOT FOR OPHTHALMIC USE. KEEP CONTAINER TIGHTLY CLOSED.**<br>NET WT 30 grams |

**13.** How many milligrams of fluocinonide are in three tubes of this cream?

**14.** What would be the percent strength of fluocinonide in a cream prepared by mixing a tube of this cream with 60 grams of a cream containing no fluocinonide?

**15.** In °C, what temperature is considered above to be "excessive heat"?

**For events 16–19:**

| PLEASE USE BALL POINT PEN – PRESS FIRMLY |
|---|

GOODTECH MEMORIAL HOSPITAL — WRITE OR IMPRINT PATIENT INFORMATION BELOW

GENERIC EQUIVALENT MAY BE DISPENSED UNLESS CHECKED ☐

| DATE | HOUR | PHYSICIANS ORDERS | DO NOT USE THIS SHEET UNLESS RED NUMBERS SHOWS | ① |
|---|---|---|---|---|
| 4/1/05 | 1735 | Vitals q/hr<br>Seizure precautions<br>Begin MgSO4 infusion at 4gm/hr and cont.<br>for 24 hours<br>SMA 7, Mg++ in AM | | |

Minnie Goodtech MD

**16.** You are directed to mix 20 g of $MgSO_4$ in 500 mL of $D_5W$. The $MgSO_4$ is supplied in 2-mL vials of 50% solution.

How many vials are needed to prepare the 500-mL order?
(NOTE: Volume adjusted to 500 mL.)

**17.** At what rate will the nurse set the infusion pump to provide the ordered dose of magnesium sulfate?

**18.** What is the drip rate in drops per minute if the infusion set delivers 20 gtt/mL?

**19.** To be prepared to supply the entire order, how many bags are needed?

**For events 20 & 21:**

**ROCEPHIN**® (ceftriaxone sodium) FOR INJECTION

**500 mg**    Single Use Vials

**Directions for Use:**
**For I.M. Administration:** Reconstitute with 1.0 mL 1% Lidocaine Hydrochloride Injection (USP) or Sterile Water for Injection (USP). Each 1 mL of solution contains approximately 350 mg equivalent of ceftriaxone.
**For I.V. Administration:** Reconstitute with 4.8 mL of an I.V. diluent specified in the accompanying package insert. Each 1 mL of solution contains approximately 100 mg equivalent of ceftriaxone.
**Withdraw entire** contents and dilute to the desired concentration with the appropriate I.V. diluent.
**Storage Prior to Reconstitution:** Store powder at room temperature 77° F (25° C) or below.
**Protect From Light.**
**Storage After Reconstitution:** See package insert.
USUAL DOSAGE: For dosage recommendations and other important prescribing information, read accompanying insert.
**ROCHE LABORATORIES INC.,** Nutley, New Jersey 07110

**20.** What is the dry powder volume of ceftriaxone sodium based on the directions for ............................... administration?

**21.** According to the directions for IM administration, how many milliliters of the reconstituted solution would provide a 200-mg dose of Rocephin®?

**For events 22–24:**

**Acyclovir Stick with Sunscreen**

℞ *(For five 5-g tubes)*

| | |
|---|---|
| Acyclovir 200-mg capsules | 5 capsules |
| Para-aminobenzoic acid | 150 mg |
| Silica gel, micronized | 120 mg |
| Polyethylene glycol 3350 | 6.5 g |
| Polyethylene glycol 300 | 15 mL |

Courtesy of *International Journal of Pharmaceutical Compounding*

**22.** How many grams of acyclovir would be required to prepare 10 tubes?

**23.** How many grams of para-aminobenzoic acid are in each tube?

**24.** How many milligrams of silica gel are in 1 gram of this formulation?

**For events 25 & 26:**

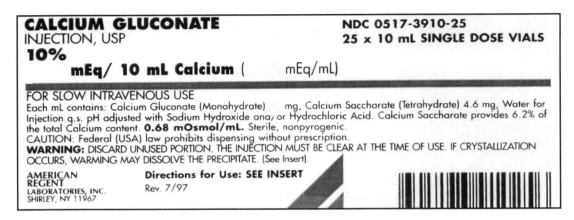

**CALCIUM GLUCONATE**
INJECTION, USP
**10%**
NDC 0517-3910-25
25 x 10 mL SINGLE DOSE VIALS

mEq/ 10 mL Calcium (          mEq/mL)

FOR SLOW INTRAVENOUS USE
Each mL contains: Calcium Gluconate (Monohydrate)     mg, Calcium Saccharate (Tetrahydrate) 4.6 mg, Water for Injection q.s. pH adjusted with Sodium Hydroxide ana/ or Hydrochloric Acid. Calcium Saccharate provides 6.2% of the total Calcium content. **0.68 mOsmol/mL.** Sterile, nonpyrogenic.
CAUTION: Federal (USA) law prohibits dispensing without prescription.
**WARNING:** DISCARD UNUSED PORTION. THE INJECTION MUST BE CLEAR AT THE TIME OF USE. IF CRYSTALLIZATION OCCURS, WARMING MAY DISSOLVE THE PRECIPITATE. (See Insert).

AMERICAN
REGENT
LABORATORIES, INC.
SHIRLEY, NY 11967

**Directions for Use: SEE INSERT**
Rev. 7/97

**25.** How many milliequivalents of calcium are contained in a vial if calcium gluconate has a molecular weight of 430 and a valence of 2?

**26.** How many milligrams of calcium gluconate are in all the vials in this package of single-dose vials?

**For events 27 & 28:**

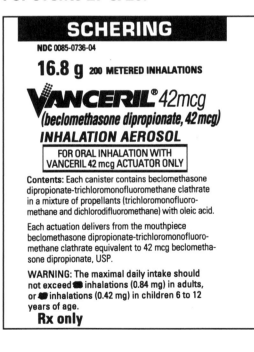

**SCHERING**

NDC 0085-0736-04

**16.8 g** 200 METERED INHALATIONS

**VANCERIL® 42mcg**
**(beclomethasone dipropionate, 42 mcg)**
**INHALATION AEROSOL**

FOR ORAL INHALATION WITH
VANCERIL 42 mcg ACTUATOR ONLY

**Contents:** Each canister contains beclomethasone dipropionate-trichloromonofluoromethane clathrate in a mixture of propellants (trichloromonofluoromethane and dichlorodifluoromethane) with oleic acid.

Each actuation delivers from the mouthpiece beclomethasone dipropionate-trichloromonofluoromethane clathrate equivalent to 42 mcg beclomethasone dipropionate, USP.

**WARNING:** The maximal daily intake should not exceed ● inhalations (0.84 mg) in adults, or ● inhalations (0.42 mg) in children 6 to 12 years of age.
**Rx only**

**27.** How many inhalations are considered maximal for an adult?

**28.** What is the mg% strength of beclomethasone in Vanceril® aerosol?

**For events 29–31:**

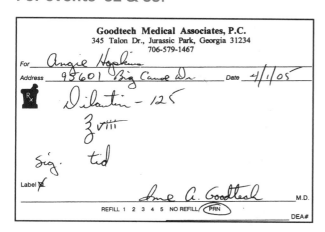

**Progesterone 50-mg/mL Topical Gel**

Rx

| | |
|---|---|
| Progesterone, micronized | 5 g |
| Hydroxyethylcellulose | 3 g |
| Alcohol, 95% | 35 mL |
| Purified water        qs | 100 mL |

Courtesy of *International Journal of Pharmaceutical Compounding*

**29.** What is the percent alcohol in the final product?

**30.** What is the percent progesterone in 1 tablespoonful of this gel?

**31.** How many grams of hydroxyethylcellulose would be required to prepare 4 fluid ounces of this gel?

**For events 32 & 33:**

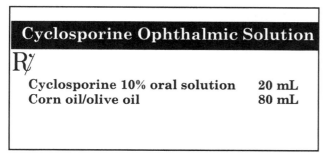

Goodtech Medical Associates, P.C.
345 Talon Dr., Jurassic Park, Georgia 31234
706-579-1467

For Angie Hopkins
Address 95601 Big Canoe Dr.     Date 4/1/05

Rx
Dilantin – 125
℥ viii
Sig.    tid
Label

Ame A. Goodtech    M.D.
REFILL 1 2 3 4 5 NO REFILL PRN
DEA#

**32.** Dr. Goodtech wants Angie to receive the Dilantin® in a dosage of 5 mg/kg/day in three equally divided doses. How many milliliters would Angie receive per dose if she weighs 66 lb and the Dilantin-125 suspension contains 125 mg of phenytoin per teaspoon?

**33.** Based on the information in event 32, how many days will the bottle last?

**For events 34–36:**

**Cyclosporine Ophthalmic Solution**

Rx

| | |
|---|---|
| Cyclosporine 10% oral solution | 20 mL |
| Corn oil/olive oil | 80 mL |

Courtesy of *International Journal of Pharmaceutical Compounding*

**34.** What is the percent strength of cyclosporine in this product?

**35.** How many milliliters of cyclosporine would be required to prepare 2 fluid ounces of this formulation?

**36.** How many milligrams of cyclosporine are in 1 mL of this formulation?

**For events 37 & 38:**

Case:

A patient named Ace Goodtech purchases a triamcinolone acetonide aerosol inhaler for $68.85. The physician has directed Ace to use 2 inhalations 3 times a day. The label on the product indicates it is a 20-g inhaler and contains 240 metered actuations. Ace is leaving town today on a two-week vacation.

**37.** How many inhalations will Ace use while he is on vacation, assuming he complies with his physician's directions?

**38.** What will be the cost for the amount of medication Ace will inhale while on vacation?

**For events 39 & 40:**

**Prior to Reconstitution:** Store at a Controlled Room Temperature 20° to 25°C ( °to °F.) Protect from light.

**After Reconstitution:** *Kefzol* is stable for 24 hours at room temperature
**Usual Adult Dose:** 250 mg to 1 gram every 6 to 8 hours.
To prepare I.V. solution - See accompanying prescribing information for directions. Each ADD-Vantage® Vial contains: 1 gram of cefazolin. The sodium content is 48 mg per gram of cefazolin.
For use only with ADD-Vantage® Flexible Diluent Container.
ADD-Vantage® (Vials and diluent containers, Abbott Laboratories )
R/only

**39.** What is the temperature range in °F for storage of Kefzol®?

**40.** How many milliequivalents of sodium will a patient receive in 3 days from Kefzol if he takes 1 gram of Kefzol q.8h? (AW sodium = 23, valence = 1)

**For events 41–44:**

| ADULT PARENTERAL NUTRITION ORDERS | | | | | ADDRESSOGRAPH | |
|---|---|---|---|---|---|---|

** ALL TPN ORDERS MUST BE IN THE PHARMACY BY 2:00 P.M. DAILY.
VOLUMES ORDERED WILL BE INFUSED OVER 24 HOURS.

1)    CONSULT NUTRITIONAL SUPPORT SERVICE

| 2) Check formulation desired: | *STANDARD CENTRAL | MODIFIED CENTRAL | **STANDARD PERIPHERAL | MODIFIED ERIPHERAL | *Standard Central formulation contains: |
|---|---|---|---|---|---|
| | ___ | ___ | ___ | ___ | 70gms protein, 420 gm dextrose, 1708 kcals excluding lipids |
| AMINO ACIDS | 70 gms | | 70 gms | | |
| DEXTROSE | 420 gms | | 140 gms | | (NOTE:Day 1 formulation will contain 210gms |
| VOLUME (mls) | 1500 mls | | 2000 mls | | dextrose & 994 kcals) rate= |
| NaCl | | | 40 mEq | | 62ml/hr Na 99mEq, Cl 98mEq, K |
| (Na) Phosphate | 18 mM | | 9 mM | | 70mEq,Ca 14mEq, Mg 24mEq, PO4 |
| Na Acetate | 75 mEq | | 70 mEq | | 18mM, Acetate 135mEq |
| KCl | 70 mEq | | 40 mEq | | |
| (K) Phosphate | | | | | **Standard Peripheral formulation |
| K Acetate | | | | | contains:  70gms protein, 140gms |
| Ca Gluconate | 14 mEq | | 7 mEq | | dextrose 686 kcals excluding |
| Mg Sulfate | 24 mEq | | 10 mEq | | lipids. rate=84ml/hr Na |
| MVI-12 | 10 mls | | 10 mls | | 122mEq, Cl 108mEq K 40mEq, Mg |
| M.T.E.-4 | 3 mls | | 3 mls | | 10mEq, PO4 9mM, Acetate 131mEq |
| Vitamin K | 1 mg | | 1 mg | | |
| Other | | | | | |

**41.** How many milliliters of an 8.5% amino acid solution is required to provide the amino acids for a standard central TPN order?

**42.** If the dextrose in the standard central TPN is provided by 600 mL of a dextrose solution, what is the percent strength of the 600 mL of dextrose?

**43.** How many milligrams of calcium gluconate (MW = 430, valence = 2) are required to prepare a standard peripheral TPN?

**44.** How many milliliters of a 1-g/10-mL calcium gluconate solution would provide the calcium gluconate needed for event 43?

**For events 45–47:**

| *(For 100 g)* | 2% | 3% |
|---|---|---|
| **Testosterone Propionate Gel** | | |
| Testosterone propionate | 2 g | 3 g |
| Mineral oil, light | 10 g | 10 g |
| Polysorbate 80 | 1 g | 1 g |
| Methylcellulose 2% gel | 87 g | 86 g |

Courtesy of *International Journal of Pharmaceutical Compounding*

**45.** How many grams of testosterone would be required to prepare 1 lb of the 3% gel?

**46.** What is the percent strength of methylcellulose in the 2% formulation?

**47.** How many milliliters of light mineral oil (sp gr 0.84) would provide the weight ordered in either of the formulas?

**For events 48 & 49:**

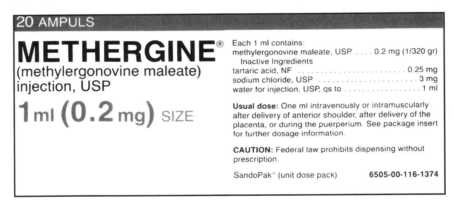

**20 AMPULS**

**METHERGINE®**
(methylergonovine maleate)
injection, USP

**1** ml **(0.2** mg) SIZE

Each 1 ml contains:
methylergonovine maleate, USP . . . . 0.2 mg (1/320 gr)
  Inactive Ingredients
tartaric acid, NF . . . . . . . . . . . . . . . . . . . . . . 0.25 mg
sodium chloride, USP . . . . . . . . . . . . . . . . . . . . 3 mg
water for injection, USP, qs to . . . . . . . . . . . . . . 1 ml

**Usual dose:** One ml intravenously or intramuscularly after delivery of anterior shoulder, after delivery of the placenta, or during the puerperium. See package insert for further dosage information.

**CAUTION:** Federal law prohibits dispensing without prescription.

SandoPak® (unit dose pack)          6505-00-116-1374

**48.** How many micrograms of tartaric acid would be in three doses of Methergine®?

**49.** How many milliequivalents of sodium chloride would be contained in all of the ampules in this package? (MW NaCl = 58.5, valence = 1)

**For events 50 & 51:**

INDICATIONS: Helps treat and prevent diaper rash. Protects chafed skin due to diaper rash and helps protect from wetness. Also helps to prevent and temporarily protect chafed, chapped, cracked, or windburned skin and lips.
DIRECTIONS: Change wet and soiled diapers promptly, cleanse the diaper area, and allow to dry. Apply **DIAPER RASH Ointment** liberally as often as necessary, with each diaper change, especially at bedtime or anytime when exposure to wet diapers may be prolonged.
ACTIVE INGREDIENT: Zinc Oxide 40%.
INACTIVE INGREDIENTS: Cod Liver Oil (High in Vitamins A & D), Petrolatum, BHA, Fragrance, Lanolin, Methylparaben, Talcum, and Purified Water.

# DIAPER RASH OINTMENT
NDC 45802-179-44
### A RECOMMENDED DIAPER RASH FORMULA AND SKIN PROTECTANT
PROTECTS SKIN, RELIEVES CHAFING
**NET WT. 4 OZ. (113 g)**

**50.** How many kilograms of zinc oxide would the manufacturer need to prepare 1000 lb of this diaper rash ointment?

**51.** The pricing code at this pharmacy puts the cost of the product on the second line of the pricing label and leaves out the decimal places. The cost of this diaper rash ointment is 104, or $1.04. What is the percent markup based on cost if the retail price to customers is $1.50?

**For events 52–54:**

### Nystatin Popsicles®

℞ *(For 10 popsicles®)*

| Nystatin powder | 2,500,000 units |
|---|---|
| Sorbitol 70% solution | 20 mL |
| Syrup, NF | 50 mL |
| Flavoring (banana, or other flavor to taste) | 5 mL |
| Purified water    qs | 300 mL |

Courtesy of *International Journal of Pharmaceutical Compounding*

**52.** What is the percent sorbitol in the final solution?

**53.** What is the percent volume-volume of the banana flavoring?

**54.** How many units of nystatin are in 2½ popsicles?

**For events 55–57:**

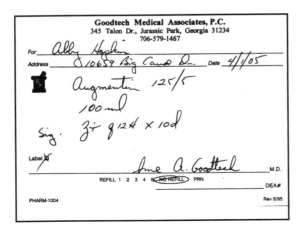

**55.** The label on the bottle of Augmentin® says to reconstitute with 90 mL of water. What is the dry powder volume displacement?

**56.** If you accidentally reconstituted this prescription with 100 mL of water, how many milliliters of the incorrectly reconstituted Augmentin would provide the appropriate dose?

(NOTE: In real life, you would probably pour this mistake down the sink and start over.)

**57.** Approximately how many pounds does Abby weigh if the package insert for Augmentin recommends a dose of 30 mg/kg/day?

**For events 58 & 59:**

50 ampuls 2 mL each    NDC 0173-0260-35

# LANOXIN® (digoxin) Injection

**500 mcg (0.5 mg) in 2 mL (250 mcg [0.25 mg] per mL)**

Store at 25°C (77°F); excursions permitted to 15 to 30°C (59 to 86°F) [see USP Controlled Room Temperature] and protect from light.

**58.** A physician orders a loading dose of digoxin to be 250 mcg I.V. q.6h for 1 day. How many single-dose ampules will be required?

**59.** A physician orders an IV digitalizing dose of 30 mcg/kg for a 14-lb baby. How many milliliters of the Lanoxin® injection should be given?

For events 60–62:

## Veterinary Electrolyte Injection

R⁄

| | |
|---|---|
| Sodium acetate trihydrate | 4.333 g |
| Potassium chloride | 467 mg |
| Calcium chloride dihydrate | 200 mg |
| Magnesium chloride | 133 mg |
| Benzyl alcohol | 0.1 mL |
| 5% Dextrose in water | 50 mL |
| Sterile water for injection    qs | 100 mL |

Courtesy of *International Journal of Pharmaceutical Compounding*

**60.** How many milliequivalents of potassium are in this formulation? (AW potassium = 39, MW potassium chloride = 74.5, valence = 1)

**61.** What is the percent dextrose in the final solution?

**62.** How many milliequivalents of magnesium chloride are in this formulation? (MW $MgCl_2$ = 95, valence = 2)

For events 63–65:

| GOODTECH MEMORIAL HOSPITAL | WRITE OR IMPRINT PATIENT INFORMATION BELOW |
|---|---|

GENERIC EQUIVALENT MAY BE DISPENSED UNLESS CHECKED ☐

| DATE | HOUR | PHYSICIANS ORDERS | DO NOT USE THIS SHEET UNLESS RED NUMBERS SHOWS. |
|---|---|---|---|
| 4/1/05 | 1530 | 1) Obtain stat PTT, PT, CBC (if not already done) | |
| | | 2) Give Bolus dose of heparin 5000 units IV | |
| | | 3) Heparin 25,000 units in 500 ml 1/2 NS at 800 units/hr via pump. Begin infusion at same time as heparin bolus dose. | |
| | | 4) Bleeding precautions | |
| | | 5) PTT follows to heparin therapy begins | |
| | | 6) Daily CBC + PTT | |
| | | Minnie Goodtech M.D. | |

**63.** The "bolus" dose of heparin is based on 75 units/kg of body weight. How many pounds does this patient weigh?

**64.** How many milliliters per hour will be given via pump to provide the patient with the prescribed heparin infusion?

**65.** If an IV set delivers 15 gtt/mL, how many gtt/min would provide the appropriate heparin dose, assuming a pump is not available and the IV set had to be utilized?

**For events 66 & 67:**

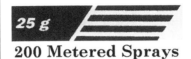

NDC 0173-0388-79

*GlaxoWellcome*

**Beconase AQ®**
*(beclomethasone dipropionate, monohydrate)*
**Nasal Spray, 0.042%***

**25 g**

**200 Metered Sprays**

Spray — For Intranasal Use Only
* Calculated on the dried basis.

Caution: Federal law prohibits dispensing without prescription.

Important: Read accompanying directions carefully.

**66.** How many milligrams of beclomethasone dipropionate are in this canister?

**67.** How many micrograms of beclomethasone dipropionate are in two intranasal sprays?

**For events 68–70:**

**Cocaine-Phenol-Tannic Acid Ointment**

Rx *(For 100 g)*

| | |
|---|---|
| Cocaine hydrochloride | 1.5 g |
| Phenol crystals | 3 g |
| Tannic acid | 10 g |
| Hydrous lanolin | 40 g |
| White petrolatum    qs | 100 g |

Courtesy of *International Journal of Pharmaceutical Compounding*

**68.** How much white petrolatum is required to prepare this product?

**69.** What is the ratio strength of cocaine in this formulation?

**70.** How many grams of phenol crystals are required to make 8 oz of this formulation?

**For events 71 & 72:**

NDC 0517 - 1130 - 01
30 mL
MULTIPLE DOSE VIAL

**EPINEPHRINE**
INJECTION, USP

FOR SC AND IM USE
FOR IV AND IC USE
AFTER DILUTION

AMERICAN
REGENT
LABORATORIES, INC.
SHIRLEY, NY 11967

Each mL contains:
1 mg Epinephrine as the hydrochloride, Water for Injection, q.s. Sodium Chloride added for isotonicity, 0.5% Chlorobutanol as a preservative and not more than 0.15% Sodium Metabisulfite as an antioxidant. pH may be adjusted with Sodium Hydroxide and/or Hydrochloric Acid.

**STORE BETWEEN 15° AND 25° C**
(59°AND 77°F).

Protect from light and freezing.
Usual Dosage: See package insert.

**71.** What is the ratio strength of this epinephrine injection?

**72.** How many milligrams of chlorobutanol are in a vial?

**For events 73 & 74:**

---

# Triple Antibiotic Ointment
(Neomycin and Polymyxin B Sulfates and
Bacitracin Zinc Ointment USP)

### First Aid Antibiotic

WARNINGS:
For external use only. Do not use in the eyes or apply over large areas of the body. In case of deep or puncture wounds, animal bites, or serious burns, consult a doctor. Stop use and consult a doctor if the condition persists or gets worse, or if a rash or other allergic reaction develops. Do not use this product if you are allergic to any of the ingredients. Do not use longer than one week unless directed by a doctor. Keep this and all drugs out of the reach of children. In case of accidental ingestion, seek professional assistance or contact a Poison Control Center immediately.

DIRECTIONS:
Clean the affected area. Apply a small amount of this product (an amount equal to the surface area of the tip of a finger) on the area 1 to 3 times daily. May be covered with a sterile bandage.

Each gram contains: neomycin sulfate 5 mg equivalent to 3.5 mg of neomycin base, polymyxin B sulfate equal to 5,000 polymyxin B units, and bacitracin zinc equal to 400 bacitracin units in a base of white petrolatum.
Store at room temperature.
See crimp of tube for Control No. & Exp. Date.

---

**73.** What is the percent markup based on selling price if the cost of this ointment is 79 cents and the retail price to customers is $1.93?

**74.** How many units of polymyxin B are in a 1-oz tube of this ointment?

**For events 75 & 76:**

---

Usual Dosage
For dosage and other prescribing information, see accompanying product literature.

Dispense in a light-resistant container as defined in the official compendium.

Store at controlled room temperature (15°-30°C, 59°-86°F). Protect from light. Do not freeze.

**Haldol®**
BRAND OF
**HALOPERIDOL INJECTION**
**(For Immediate Release)**
**5 mg per mL**
10 x 1-mL
STERILE AMPULS

Caution: Federal law prohibits dispensing without prescription.

**McNEIL PHARMACEUTICAL**

Each mL contains:
Haloperidol 5 mg
(as the lactate) with
1.8 mg methylparaben,
0.2 mg propylparaben,
and lactic acid for pH
adjustment to 3.0-3.6

For Intramuscular Use

McNeil Pharmaceutical
McNeilab, Inc.
Spring House, PA 19477
© McN '93     701-94-066-4

---

**75.** The attending physician wants his 220-lb psychotic patient to receive Haldol® 0.1 mg/kg/day in divided doses b.i.d. How many milligrams of Haldol will this patient receive per dose?

**76.** How many ampules must be sent to the patient's unit to provide a week's supply of the Haldol prescribed in event 75?

**For events 77–79:**

---

## Piroxicam 1% Alcoholic Gel

R℞  Piroxicam                              1 g
      Hydroxypropylcellulose              1.75 g
      Propylene glycol                     5 mL
      Polysorbate 80                       2 mL
      70% Isopropyl alcohol qs          100 mL

---

Courtesy of *International Journal of Pharmaceutical Compounding*

**77.** What is the weight of propylene glycol (sp gr 1.04) in this formula?

**78.** What is the percent strength of hydroxypropylcellulose in 3 quarts of this formulation?

**79.** How many grams of piroxicam are required to prepare a gallon of this formulation?

**For events 80 & 81:**

## Domeboro® ASTRINGENT SOLUTION

DOMEBORO provides soothing, effective relief of minor skin irritations. For over 50 years doctors have been recommending DOMEBORO ASTRINGENT SOLUTION to help relieve minor skin irritations.

**INDICATIONS:** For temporary relief of minor skin irritations due to poison ivy, poison oak, poison sumac, insect bites, athlete's foot or rashes caused by soaps, detergents, cosmetics or jewelry.

**DIRECTIONS:** One packet dissolved in 16 ounces of water makes a modified Burow's Solution approximately equivalent to a 1:40 dilution; two packets, a 1:20 dilution; and four packets, a 1:10 dilution. Dissolve one or two packets in water and stir the solution until fully dissolved. Do not strain or filter the solution. Can be used as a compress, wet dressing or as a soak. AS A COMPRESS OR WET DRESSING: saturate a clean, soft, white cloth (such as a diaper or torn sheet) in the solution; gently squeeze and apply loosely to the affected area. Saturate the cloth in the solution every 15 to 30 minutes and apply to affected area. Discard solution after each use. Repeat as often as necessary. AS A SOAK: soak affected area in the solution for 15 to 30 minutes. Discard solution after each use. Repeat 3 times a day.

**WARNINGS:** If condition worsens or symptoms persist for more than 7 days, discontinue use of the product and consult a doctor. For external use only. Avoid contact with the eyes. Do not cover compress or wet dressing with plastic to prevent evaporation. Keep this and all drugs out of the reach of children. In case of accidental ingestion, seek professional assistance or contact a Poison Control Center immediately.

**ACTIVE INGREDIENTS:** Each powder packet, when dissolved in water and ready to use, provides the active ingredient aluminum acetate resulting from the reaction of calcium acetate 938 mg, and aluminum sulfate 1191 mg. The resulting astringent solution is buffered to an acid pH.

**INACTIVE INGREDIENT:** Dextrin

PROOF OF PURCHASE
UNIVERSAL PRODUCT CODE (UPC)

MADE IN USA

Questions or Comments
Call 1-800-800-4793
8:30–5:00 EST M–F

Bayer ⊕  Bayer Corporation
          Consumer Care Division
          Elkhart, IN 46515 USA

0  16500 02324  1

**80.** What is the percent strength of the Domeboro® dilution when 1 packet is dissolved in a pint of water?

**81.** How many Domeboro packets will a patient need if he is preparing 1 pint of the 1:20 dilution q.i.d. × 5 days?

**For events 82 & 83:**

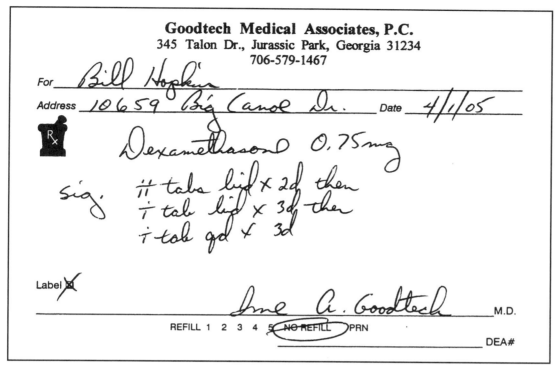

82. How many dexamethasone 0.75-mg tablets should be dispensed to properly fill this prescription?

83. How many total grams of dexamethasone will this patient receive?

**For events 84 & 85:**

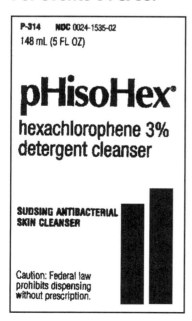

84. How many grams of hexachlorophene are in a bottle of pHisoHex®?

85. How many kilograms of hexachlorophene would be required to prepare a 20,000-liter vat of pHisoHex?

**For events 86–88:**

---

## Idoxuridine Ophthalmic Solution

R℞

| | | |
|---|---|---|
| Idoxuridine | | 100 mg |
| Thimerosal | | 2 mg |
| Sterile water for injection | qs | 100 mL |

---

Courtesy of *International Journal of Pharmaceutical Compounding*

**86.** What is the percent strength of idoxuridine in this formulation?

**87.** What is the milligram percent of thimerosal in this formulation?

**88.** How many micrograms of idoxuridine would be required to prepare ½ fluid ounce of this formulation?

**For events 89 & 90:**

NDC 0456-0672-99

**7g** 100 metered inhalations

**AEROBID**®
(flunisolide)
**Inhaler System**

FOR ORAL INHALATION ONLY

**Contains** flunisolide as the hemihydrate suspended in propellants (trichloromono-fluoromethane, dichlorodifluoromethane and dichlorotetrafluoroethane) with sorbitan trioleate as a dispersing agent.
Each activation delivers approximately 250 mcg flunisolide to the patient.
**Caution:** Federal law prohibits dispensing without prescription.

mfd for

 **FOREST PHARMACEUTICALS, INC.**
SUBSIDIARY OF FOREST LABORATORIES, INC.
ST. LOUIS, MISSOURI 63045

**89.** The recommended dose for Aerobid® is 2 inhalations b.i.d. How many canisters should a patient purchase if he is going on a trip around the world that will last 92 days?

**90.** How many milligrams of flunisolide will the patient inhale during the trip around the world mentioned in event 89?

**For events 91–94:**

GOODTECH MEMORIAL HOSPITAL

WRITE OR IMPRINT PATIENT INFORMATION BELOW

GENERIC EQUIVALENT MAY BE DISPENSED UNLESS CHECKED ☐

| DATE | HOUR | PHYSICIANS ORDERS | DO NOT USE THIS SHEET UNLESS RED NUMBERS SHOWS. |
|------|------|-------------------|-----------------|
| 4/1/05 | 0800 | Admit to Dr. Goodtech's service | |
| | | Dx: pneumonia, N/V | |
| | | CBC č diff, SMA 7 in AM | |
| | | Zosyn 3 gm IV q6h | |
| | | Solu-Medrol 80mg IV q6h | |
| | | Reglan 10-20 mg IV q6h prn N/V | |
| | | Tylenol 325mg ī-īī po q4-6h prn pain/HA | |
| | | Regular diet | |
| | | | Minnie Goodtech MD |

91. Solu-Medrol® is available for injection in a 125-mg/2-mL vial. How many milliliters of this injection are required for each ordered dose?

92. Reglan® injection is available in 2-mL ampules containing 5 mg/mL. How many ampules would supply the maximum ordered daily dose?

93. How many grams of Tylenol® would this patient receive daily if he received the maximum quantity ordered?

94. Zosyn® is reconstituted in the pharmacy to contain 3.375 g/20 mL. How many milliliters should be administered every 6 hours according to Dr. Minnie Goodtech's order to provide this patient an unusual dose?

**For events 95–97:**

| | | | | |
|---|---|---|---|---|
| 58-0789 -R5-Rev. June, 1999 | | | | |

Recommended dosage for adults with heart block, Adams-Stokes attacks, and cardiac arrent:

| Route of Administration | Preparation of Dilution | Initial Dose | Subsequent Dose Range* |
|---|---|---|---|
| Bolus intravenous injection | Dilute 1 mL (0.2 mg) to 10 mL with Sodium Chloride Injection, USP, or 5% Dextrose Injection, USP | ___ mg to ___ mg (1 mL to 3 mL of diluted solution) | ___ mg to ___ mg (0.5 mL to 10 mL of diluted solution) |
| Intravenous infusion | Dilute 10 mL (2 mg) in 500 mL of 5% Dextrose Injection, USP | 5 mcg/min. ___ mL of diluted solution per minute) | |
| Intramuscular | Use Solution 1:5000 undiluted | 0.2 mg | 0.02 mg to 1 mg ( ___ mL to ___ mL) |

**ᵃ ISUPREL®**
**|||** Isoproterenol Hydrochloride Injection, USP

**Sterile Injection 1:5000**

95. What is the range in milligrams of Isuprel® that a patient would receive as an initial dose from a bolus intravenous injection route of administration?

96. How many milliliters per minute of the diluted Isuprel solution would provide the initial dose from an intravenous infusion route of administration?

97. How many milliliters of undiluted Isuprel would provide the initial dose by the intramuscular route of administration?

**For events 98 & 99:**

| **Analgesic Medication Stick** | |
|---|---|
| ℞ *(For 100 g)* | |
| Methyl salicylate | 35 g |
| Menthol | 15 g |
| Sodium stearate | 13 g |
| Purified water | 12 g |
| Propylene glycol | 25 g |

Courtesy of *International Journal of Pharmaceutical Compounding*

98. What is the ratio strength of propylene glycol in this formulation?

99. How many grams of sodium stearate are needed to make 2.75 kg of this formulation?

**For events 100 & 101 (our bonus question):**

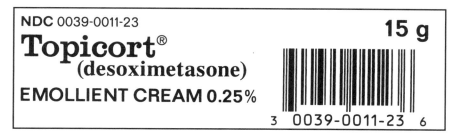

6505-00-926-2095

# fougera

## HYDROCORTISONE
## CREAM, U.S.P. 1%

CONTAINS: 10 mg of Hydrocortisone per gram in a base containing Glyceryl Monostearate, Polyoxyl 40 Stearate, Glycerin, Paraffin, Stearyl Alcohol, Isopropyl Palmitate, Sorbitan Monostearate, Benzyl Alcohol, Potassium Sorbate, Lactic Acid, and Purified Water.

NET WT. 1 OZ. (28.35g)

NDC 0039-0011-23

# Topicort®
### (desoximetasone)

EMOLLIENT CREAM 0.25%

15 g

3  0039-0011-23  6

**100.** How many grams of 2.5% hydrocortisone cream should be mixed with this tube of hydrocortisone to prepare a 1.25% hydrocortisone cream?

## *BONUS (THIS IS REAL TRICKY!)*

**101.** What would be the percent strength of desoximetasone in a product prepared by mixing the tubes of hydrocortisone and Topicort®?

# Posttest II: Standardized Test Preparation

Throughout this book, you have encountered hundreds of practice problems requiring fill-in-the-blank answers. Most standardized exams for certifications will make it easier for you by asking multiple-choice questions, which you have likely been exposed to multiple times in school. The important point to realize when answering these questions is that the writers will frequently give incorrect choices that can be numbers you may select carelessly. For example: How many milligrams will a 100-pound patient receive if the dose is 8 mcg per pound? You will perform a ratio and proportion calculation and come up with an answer of 800 mcg. One of the choices for this multiple choice question will be "800," and many test takers will jump all over this choice. Upon further review, however, you will see that the correct answer is "0.8," because you were asked to answer in milligrams and not micrograms. Hopefully, the following multiple choice items will help you fine-tune your skills and prepare you for any standardized exams you may encounter. **Caution:** I will continually try to trick you on these questions, so be prepared, read carefully, and don't allow me to trap you. **GOOD LUCK!!!**

**(For questions 1–5)**

1. You receive the following prescription to be compounded:

   RX
   
        Fluticasone Propionate 0.005% ointment .............. 15g
        Triamcinolone Acetonide 0.1% ointment................. 80g
        Petrolatum Ointment................................ q.s. ad 180g
   Sig. Apply as directed

   How many grams of petrolatum are required to compound this prescription?

   a. 15
   b. 85
   c. 165
   d. 180
   e. Cannot be calculated with the information provided

2. What is the percent strength of triamcinolone in the final product?

   a. 0.044
   b. 0.44
   c. 4.4
   d. 44
   e. More than 50

3. What is the percent strength of triamcinolone in 10 grains of the final product?

   a. 0.044
   b. 0.28
   c. 0.89
   d. 2.56
   e. More than 3

4. What would be the final weight in grams of the compounded prescription if the abbreviations "q.s." and "ad" were omitted?

   a. 95
   b. 120
   c. 180
   d. 240
   e. 275

5. What would be the percent fluticasone in the product if the abbreviations "q.s." and "ad" were omitted?

   a. 0.00027
   b. 0.005
   c. 0.027
   d. 0.5
   e. Greater than 1

**(For questions 6–8)**

6. A mixture of dopamine 800 mg in 500 mL of NS would produce a dopamine concentration of how many micrograms per milliliter?

   a. 0.16
   b. 1.6
   c. 16
   d. 160
   e. 1600

7. How many 40 mg/mL vials of dopamine would be required to prepare a liter of this solution if each vial contained 10 mL?

   a. 0.2
   b. 0.4
   c. 2
   d. 4
   e. Not enough information provided to calculate the number of vials

8. How many milliliters of the solution in question 6 would provide a 3000-mcg/min dose of dopamine for an hour?

   a. 1.87
   b. 11.3
   c. 56.5
   d. 112.5
   e. More than 150

**(For questions 9 & 10)**

9. How many milliliters of a 3 g/15 mL stock solution would provide a 300-mg dose?

   a. 0.015
   b. 0.15
   c. 1.5
   d. 15
   e. 150

10. What is the percent strength of this stock solution?

    a. 0.02
    b. 0.2
    c. 2
    d. 20
    e. Less than 0.02

**(For questions 11 & 12)**

**11.** How many fluid ounces would need to be dispensed to provide a patient a 1.5-tbsp dose of a drug q.i.d. × 2 days?

    a. 1
    b. 4
    c. 6
    d. 30
    e. 180

**12.** What percent of a 1-pint stock bottle of the drug would remain after dispensing the prescription in question 11?

    a. 0.375
    b. 0.625
    c. 37.5
    d. 62.5
    e. More than 75

**(For questions 13 & 14)**

**13.** How many methylprednisolone 4-mg tablets would be needed to fill a prescription with the following directions?

Day 1: 2 tablets at breakfast, 1 at lunch, 1 at dinner, and 2 at bedtime
Day 2: 1 tablet at breakfast, 1 at lunch, 1 at dinner, and 2 at bedtime
Day 3: 1 tablet at breakfast, 1 at lunch, 1 at dinner, and 1 at bedtime
Day 4: 1 tablet at breakfast, 1 at lunch, and 1 at bedtime
Day 5: 1 tablet at breakfast and 1 at bedtime
Day 6: 1 tablet at breakfast

    a. 19
    b. 20
    c. 21
    d. 22
    e. 23

**14.** How many grams of methylprednisolone would the patient receive over the 6 days of therapy?

    a. 0.021
    b. 0.084
    c. 2.1
    d. 21
    e. 84

**(For questions 15 & 16)**

**15.** Enoxaparin sodium injection is available in 40 mg/0.4 mL-prefilled syringes. How many syringes would be required to provide the recommended 40-mg/day prophylactic dose for 3 weeks to 18 patients after hip replacements in an orthopedic surgery center?

a. 18
b. 21
c. 36
d. 182
e. 378

**16.** How many total combined grams of enoxaparin would the patients receive if they all completed the full course of therapy?

a. 1.512
b. 15.12
c. 151.2
d. 1512
e. 15,120

**(For questions 17 & 18)**

**17.** A patient receives a prescription for Coumadin 5 mg (scored) tablets and is instructed to take 5 mg and 7.5 mg on alternating days. How many 5-mg tablets would need to be dispensed to provide a 90-day supply?

a. 40
b. 68
c. 76
d. 113
e. More than 118

**18.** How many grams of Coumadin would this patient receive in September?

a. 0.1875
b. 1.875
c. 18.75
d. 187.5
e. 1875

**(For questions 19 & 20)**

**19.** Lanoxin pediatric elixir is available in a 0.05-mg/mL strength. A child's doctor prescribes 10 mcg/kg/day p.o. divided q.6h. What volume in milliliters of the elixir would provide a single dose for the 44-lb patient?

    a. 0.1
    b. 1
    c. 4
    d. 100
    e. 400

**20.** How many days would a 60-mL bottle last for this patient?

    a. 5
    b. 10
    c. 12
    d. 15
    e. 60

**21.** A pharmacy compounds suppositories that each have a calculated weight of 3 grams. What would be the permissible range of weights in milligrams for the suppositories if the maximum margin of error is 5%?

    a. 2850–3150
    b. 2800–3200
    c. 2750–3250
    d. 2500–3500
    e. 2350–3650

**(For questions 22 & 23)**

**22.** Lactulose is available in a 10 g/15 mL-solution, and the maximum adult dose for constipation is 4 tbsp. daily. How many milligrams of lactulose would a patient receive each day from the maximum dose?

    a. 10
    b. 40
    c. 200
    d. 20,000
    e. 40,000

**23.** How many pints would be required to provide a 30-day supply of the maximum dose of lactulose?

a. 0.00375
b. 0.0375
c. 0.375
d. 3.75
e. 37.5

**(For questions 24 & 25)**

**24.** How many 750-mg tablets of a drug would be required to prepare a pint of a solution containing 500 mg/tsp?

a. Less than 10
b. 12
c. 34
d. 48
e. 64

**25.** What is the percent strength of the solution in question 24?

a. 0.05
b. 0.1
c. 0.5
d. 10
e. 50

**(For questions 26 & 27)**

**26.** A physician orders cefazolin sodium for a 7-year-old child in a dosage of 40 mg/kg/day divided equally into three doses. How many milligrams would a 66-lb child receive per dose?

a. 40
b. 120
c. 400
d. 1200
e. 4000

**27.** How many grams of cefazolin would the child in question 26 receive over a 2-week course of therapy?

a. 5.6
b. 16.8
c. 560
d. 5600
e. 16,800

**(For questions 28 & 29)**

**28.** A medication order for amoxicillin 500 mg instructs a patient to take 2 capsules b.i.d. × 2 days and then 1 capsule t.i.d. × 10 days. How many capsules would be required to fill this order?

    a. 30
    b. 34
    c. 38
    d. 42
    e. 64

**29.** How many grams of amoxicillin would the patient in question 28 receive in the first week of therapy?

    a. Less than 10
    b. 10.5
    c. 11.5
    d. 10,500
    e. 11,500

**(For questions 30 & 31)**

**30.** A dosing regimen for ifosfamide is 1200 $mg/m^2$/day for 5 days, every 3 weeks for 4 cycles. How many milligrams would a 187-lb patient with a body surface area (BSA) of 1.9 $m^2$ receive daily?

    a. 2280
    b. 4320
    c. 5565
    d. 11,400
    e. More than 15,000

**31.** How many grams of ifosfamide would the patient in question 30 receive in all 4 cycles?

    a. 9.12
    b. 11.4
    c. 45.6
    d. 11,400
    e. More than 42,000

**32.** How many milligrams of benzalkonium chloride should be used to prepare a gallon of 1:4000 solution?

    a. 0.096
    b. 0.96
    c. 9.6
    d. 96
    e. 960

**(For questions 33 & 34)**

**33.** How many milliliters of 8% Burow's solution and 20% Burow's solution should be mixed to prepare a liter of 15% Burow's solution?

    a. 583 mL of 20% and 417 mL of 8%
    b. 417 mL of 20% and 583 mL of 8%
    c. 385 mL of 20% and 615 mL of 8%
    d. 615 mL of 20% and 385 mL of 8%
    e. You can't add a 20% solution with an 8% solution, to get a 15% solution, because the final solution would be 28%

**34.** How many milliliters of water could be added to the 20% Burow's solution to prepare the amount of 15% Burow's solution desired in question 33?

    a. Less than 200
    b. 250
    c. 750
    d. 950
    e. You can't add water to a 20% solution to get a 15% solution . . . duh!!!

**(For questions 35 & 36)**

**35.** How many milliliters of EryPed 400 mg/5 mL would provide a patient with a 280-mg dose (calculated by patient weight)?

    a. 0.35
    b. 0.9
    c. 2.8
    d. 3.5
    e. 4.6

**36.** How many milliliters of EryPed in question 35 would be required to provide the calculated dose q.8h × 10 days?

    a. 10.5
    b. 35
    c. 55
    d. 95
    e. 105

**37.** A patient received a half liter of 10% fat emulsion four times during a hospitalization. How many grams of fat did the patient receive?

    a. 50
    b. 100
    c. 150
    d. 200
    e. 250

**(For questions 38–40)**

**38.** How many milligrams of fluorouracil would a 165-lb patient with a BSA of 1.7 m² receive on 5 successive days at a dosage rate of 14 mg/kg/day?

    a. 375
    b. 835
    c. 1050
    d. 5250
    e. 7725

**39.** How many total milliliters of 2.5 g/50 mL fluorouracil solution would be needed to provide the entire dosing regimen to the patient in question 38?

    a. 0.85
    b. 8.5
    c. 21
    d. 105
    e. 210

**40.** The physician decides to dose the patient in question 38 using BSA instead of body weight. If the recommended BSA dose is 750 mg/m²/day, how many milligrams would the patient receive daily?

    a. 228
    b. 441
    c. 850
    d. 1275
    e. 2010

**41.** A patient presents a prescription for metoprolol succinate 100 mg and is instructed to take ½ tablet b.i.d. How many tablets would provide a 3-month supply for this patient?

    a. 30
    b. 45
    c. 60
    d. 90
    e. 180

**(For questions 42–44)**

**42.** A physician orders lincomycin 800 mg IV q.8h × 7 days. This medication is available in the pharmacy in 300-mg/mL vials. How many total milliliters will be required to provide the daily dose?

    a. 2.67
    b. 4
    c. 8
    d. 18
    e. 56

**43.** How many grams of lincomycin will the patient in question 42 receive in the full course of therapy?

   a. 2.4
   b. 5.6
   c. 16.8
   d. 240
   e. 16,800

**44.** What will be the total cost of the entire regimen in question 42 if the average wholesale price (AWP) for lincomycin is $181.75 for a 10-mL vial?

   a. $48.22
   b. $145.40
   c. $339.11
   d. $829.29
   e. $1017.80

**(For questions 45–47)**

**45.** What would be the concentration in milligrams per milliliter of 4 fluid ounces of a suspension prepared with #20 250-mg paromomycin capsules?

   a. 3.2
   b. 4.9
   c. 22.2
   d. 41.7
   e. 63.8

**46.** What would be the percent strength of the paromomycin suspension in question 45?

   a. 0.0042
   b. 0.042
   c. 0.42
   d. 4.2
   e. 42

**47.** How many grams of paromomycin would be in a tablespoon of the suspension in question 45?

   a. 0.625
   b. 0.892
   c. 8.45
   d. 98.2
   e. 631

**(For questions 48–50)**

**48.** A 46-lb patient receives the following prescription:

Ampicillin 125/5
200 mL
Take 1½ teaspoonsful p.o. q.6h until gone

How many milligrams of ampicillin will the patient receive daily?

   a. 125
   b. 188
   c. 250
   d. 564
   e. 750

**49.** How many "full" doses of ampicillin will the patient receive from the volume dispensed?

   a. 6
   b. 15
   c. 22
   d. 26
   e. 27

**50.** How many milligrams of ampicillin per kilogram of body weight is the patient receiving daily?

   a. 21.2
   b. 31.8
   c. 35.7
   d. 42.6
   e. More than 50

**(For questions 51–53)**

**51.** Isoniazid 50 mg/5 mL is available as an oral syrup and is supplied in pint bottles. One of the treatment regimens carries a maximum daily dose of 300 mg. How many tablespoonsful would provide the maximum daily dose?

   a. 2
   b. 4
   c. 6
   d. 8
   e. 10

**52.** How many pints would be required to provide the maximum daily dose of isoniazid for 9 months of therapy?

    a. 3
    b. 5
    c. 14
    d. 17
    e. 21

**53.** How much would 1 week of therapy of isoniazid in question 51 cost if the AWP was $0.86/mL?

    a. Less than $10
    b. $25.80
    c. $88.87
    d. $180.60
    e. More than $235

**(For questions 54 & 55)**

**54.** An order is received to add 2000 mg of magnesium sulfate to an IV solution. How many milliliters of a 50% magnesium sulfate solution will be needed?

    a. 2
    b. 4
    c. 6
    d. 8
    e. More than 10

**55.** If 1 gram of magnesium sulfate equals 98.6 mg of elemental magnesium, how many grams of elemental magnesium are represented in this IV order?

    a. 0.197
    b. 0.54
    c. 2.01
    d. 195
    e. 222

**(For questions 56 & 57)**

**56.** How many grams of ointment base would need to be mixed with 15 g of mometasone ointment 0.1% to reduce the strength of the ointment to 0.025%?

   a. 15
   b. 30
   c. 45
   d. 60
   e. Can't be done

**57.** How many milligrams of mometasone ointment 0.1% would need to be added to 30 mg of mometasone ointment 0.1% to increase the strength to 0.3%?

   a. 30
   b. 60
   c. 90
   d. 120
   e. Can't be done

**(For questions 58–60)**

**58.** Gentamicin is available as a 40-mg/mL injection. How many milliliters would be required to compound 120 mL of a solution containing 1 mg/mL?

   a. 3
   b. 5
   c. 17
   d. 30
   e. 50

**59.** What would be the percent strength of the 120-mL solution in question 58?

   a. 0.1
   b. 2
   c. 10
   d. 40
   e. 100

**60.** How many 2-mL vials of gentamicin 40 mg/mL injection would be needed to prepare the 120-mL solution?

   a. 0.5
   b. 1.5
   c. 2.5
   d. 3.5
   e. More than 4

**(For questions 61–63)**

**61.** A veterinarian wrote the following prescription to be compounded for a horse:

RX

    Hydrocortisone Powder............................................. 2%
    Menthol................................................................ 0.5%
    Lubriderm Lotion...............................................ad 1 pint
Sig: Apply 15 mL topically b.i.d.

How many milligrams of hydrocortisone powder will be needed to compound this prescription?

a. 0.96
b. 9.6
c. 96
d. 960
e. 9600

**62.** How many grams of menthol are required to prepare this prescription?

a. 0.24
b. 2.4
c. 24
d. 240
e. 2400

**63.** How many days will this prescription last?

a. 4
b. 8
c. 12
d. 16
e. More than 18

**(For questions 64–66)**

**64.** A pharmacy receives an order to compound 6 fluid ounces of a solution to contain 2.5 mcg/mL of a medication. How many 0.05-mg tablets of the medication would be needed to prepare this order?

a. 0.009
b. 0.09
c. 0.9
d. 9
e. More than 90

**65.** How many grams of medication would be in 2 tsp of this solution?

    a. 0.000025
    b. 0.00025
    c. 0.0025
    d. 0.025
    e. 0.25

**66.** How many days would this compounded solution last if the patient received 75 mcg b.i.d.?

    a. 2
    b. 3
    c. 4
    d. 5
    e. More than 6

**(For questions 67–70)**

**67.** A manufacturer prepares a 2500-pound batch of 1.5% hydrocortisone cream each month. How many kilograms of hydrocortisone are needed to prepare a single batch?

    a. 1.7025
    b. 17.025
    c. 170.25
    d. 1702.5
    e. 17,025

**68.** What would be the resulting percent strength if the manufacturer recklessly used 71 kg of hydrocortisone to prepare a batch?

    a. Less than 5
    b. 6.25
    c. 8.75
    d. 35.83
    e. More than 40

**69.** How many 120-g tubes of 1.5% ointment can be filled from a batch?

    a. Less than 1000
    b. 2367
    c. 7993
    d. 9458
    e. More than 10,000

**70.** A 120-g tube sells for $46.85, and a patient applies 1 g topically t.i.d. What is the daily cost of the medication for the patient?

a. $0.39
b. $0.92
c. $1.17
d. $3.85
e. $4.11

**(For questions 71 & 72)**

**71.** Sodium bicarbonate 8.4% is available in 50-mL vials. How many milligrams of sodium bicarbonate are in each vial?

a. 4.2
b. 42
c. 420
d. 4200
e. 42,000

**72.** How many milligrams per milliliter would be in 1 gallon of sodium bicarbonate solution?

a. Less than 0.0084
b. 0.084
c. 8.4
d. 84
e. More than 840

**(For questions 73 & 74)**

**73.** A patient purchases a pint bottle of potassium chloride 20% solution. How many milligrams of potassium chloride would the patient receive daily if the patient took 1 teaspoonful t.i.d.?

a. 1
b. 3
c. 100
d. 1000
e. 3000

**74.** There are 74.5 mg in each milliequivalent of potassium chloride. How many milliequivalents of potassium chloride would this patient receive daily?

a. 3.9
b. 40.3
c. 72.8
d. 103.6
e. More than 175

**(For questions 75 & 76)**

**75.** A pharmacy purchased 2 gallons of a cough syrup and repackaged the liquid in 4-fluid-ounce bottles for resale. Approximately how many bottles were filled?

a. Less than 20
b. 32
c. 64
d. 128
e. More than 150

**76.** If the pharmacy paid a total of $135.80 for the bulk cough syrup and dispensing bottles and then sold the smaller bottles for $5.95 each, what was the final profit from the sale of all of the bottles?

a. $37
b. $114
c. $189
d. $245
e. More than $300

**(For questions 77 & 78)**

**77.** The label on an antibiotic suspension states to add 78 mL of water to yield 100 mL of 400 mg/5 mL suspension. How much additional water would need to be added to reduce the final strength to 200 mg/5 mL?

a. 35
b. 62
c. 78
d. 100
e. None of the above

**78.** What would be the concentration in milligrams per milliliter if a mistake was made in preparing the original bottle and 118 mL of water was added instead of 78?

a. 17.27
b. 23.86
c. 57.14
d. 285.31
e. 332.43

**79.** Scopolamine injection is available in a 0.4 mg/mL strength and has been used for sedation in a 0.3-mg dose q.i.d. How many milliliters would provide the total daily dose?

a. 2
b. 3
c. 4
d. 5
e. 6

**(For questions 80 & 81)**

**80.** How many milliliters of 10% stock solution of a chemical are needed to prepare 4 fluid ounces of a solution containing 20 mg of the chemical per milliliter?

a. 0.024
b. 0.24
c. 2.4
d. 24
e. More than 28

**81.** How many milliliters of water and 10% stock solution are required to prepare a pint of 3% solution?

a. 336 mL of water and 144 mL stock solution
b. 144 mL of water and 336 mL stock solution
c. 225 mL of water and 255 mL stock solution
d. 255 mL of water and 225 mL stock solution
e. Can't mix water with the stock solution to decrease the percent strength

**(For questions 82–84)**

**82.** RX

> Hydrocortisone Powder............................................. 1%
> Vioform Powder ...........................................................5g
> Menthol.................................................................. 0.5%
> Phenol .................................................................. 0.5%
> Cold cream........................................................ ad 180g
Sig: Apply as directed

How many grams of hydrocortisone are in the final product?

a. 1.8
b. 2.6
c. 3.4
d. 5.5
e. 17.9

**83.** What is the percent strength of vioform in the final product?

a. 0.028
b. 0.19
c. 2.23
d. 2.78
e. More than 3

**84.** How many milligrams of phenol are in the final product?

a. 0.09
b. 0.9
c. 9
d. 90
e. 900

**(For questions 85 & 86)**

**85.** A physician orders eptifibatide 180 mcg/kg STAT followed by a continuous infusion of 2 mcg/kg/min for a 210-lb, 63-year-old woman. How many milliliters of eptifibatide 2 mg/mL are required to provide the STAT dose?

a. 4.3
b. 8.6
c. 17.2
d. 41.6
e. More than 45

**86.** How many milligrams of eptifibatide will the patient receive in 1 hour from the continuous infusion?

a. 5.73
b. 11.46
c. 5760
d. 11,461
e. 57,605

**(For questions 87 & 88)**

**87.** A pharmacy purchases a bottle of 100 Toprol XL 50-mg tablets. The AWP for these tablets is $118, and the pharmacy has a purchasing contract of AWP minus 10% plus $2.75. How much does the pharmacy actually pay for the 100 tablets?

a. $78.25
b. $97.23
c. $103.87
d. $108.95
e. $112.61

**88.** How much would a prescription for Toprol XL 50 mg, 1 tablet b.i.d. × 30 days cost the pharmacy?

a. $32.69
b. $41.31
c. $47.93
d. $65.37
e. More than $68

**(For questions 89 & 90)**

**89.** The suggested maximum concentration of potassium phosphate for central line administration is 26.8 mmol potassium phosphate/100 mL (40 mEq potassium/100 mL). How many milliliters of a 45 mmol/15 mL solution of potassium phosphate would provide 100 mL of the maximum concentration?

a. 8.93
b. 11.24
c. 12.87
d. 16.79
e. 18.09

**90.** How many milliequivalents of potassium would be in a concentration of 10 mmol of potassium phosphate/100 mL?

a. 3.25
b. 7.45
c. 8.8
d. 11.5
e. 14.9

**(For questions 91 & 92)**

**91.** A 2% pilocarpine hydrochloride ophthalmic solution is available in 15-mL bottles. How many milligrams per milliliter of pilocarpine does this represent?

a. 0.2
b. 2
c. 20
d. 200
e. 2000

**92.** How many milligrams of pilocarpine would be in 4 drops if the dropper bottle delivered 20 drops/mL?

    a. 0.04
    b. 0.4
    c. 4
    d. 40
    e. 400

**(For questions 93 & 94)**

**93.** A 72-year-old patient weighs 262 lbs and is to receive theophylline by continuous infusion at a rate of 0.3 mg/kg/hr with a maximum daily dose of 400 mg unless serum levels indicate a need for larger doses. How many milligrams of theophylline will this patient receive per hour?

    a. 35.7
    b. 78.6
    c. 359
    d. 786
    e. 2142

**94.** Which of the following statements is correct?

    a. The dosing regimen exceeds the recommended maximum daily dose.
    b. The dosing regimen is safe and below the maximum daily dose.
    c. The daily dose cannot be determined from the information provided.
    d. The dose can comfortably be increased without checking serum levels.
    e. None of the above is correct.

**(For questions 95 & 96)**

**95.** A veterinarian requests that you prepare 5 fluid ounces of a tobramycin solution to contain 30 mg/mL. The only product you have available is in a 1.2 g/30 mL strength. How many milliliters of the available product will be needed to prepare the veterinarian's order?

    a. 4.5
    b. 9.1
    c. 84.4
    d. 112.5
    e. 4500

**96.** How many milliliters of diluent will need to be added to the calculated volume of tobramycin 1.2 g/30 mL to prepare the requested order?

a. 37.5
b. 46.7
c. 81.1
d. 91.3
e. 112.5

**(For questions 97–100)**

**97.** You are requested to compound 120 mL of metoclopramide suspension containing 5 mg/tbsp. How many 10-mg metoclopramide tablets will be needed?

a. 2
b. 4
c. 6
d. 9
e. 12

**98.** How many kilograms of metoclopramide will be in 2 quarts of this solution?

a. 0.00064
b. 0.0064
c. 0.64
d. 6.4
e. 640

**99.** What is the final concentration of metoclopramide in milligrams per milliliter?

a. 0.3333
b. 3.333
c. 33.33
d. 333.3
e. 3333

**100.** What is the percent strength of metoclopramide in the final solution?

a. 0.00033
b. 0.0033
c. 0.033
d. 0.33
e. 3.3

# Answer Key

## CHAPTER 1

1a   200 (rule 1)
1b   No value (rule 3)
1c   3000 (rule 1)
1d   No value (rule 2)
1e   40 (rule 4)
1f   No value (rule 6)
1g   55 (rule 5)
1h   No value (rule 8)
1i   12 (rule 5)
1j   No value (rule 7)
1k   22
1l   51
1m   110
1n   150
1o   66
1p   1004
1q   515
1r   29
1s   445
1t   No value, just seeing if you are awake.
1u   XVIII
1v   XXXIV
1w   XLVII
1x   LXII
1y   CDLXXX
1z   MCMXCIX

2a   $7 \times 1/12 = 7/1 \times 1/12 = 7/12$
2b   $3/5 \times 1/5 = 3/25$
2c   $1\,1/6 \times 2\,1/2 = 7/6 \times 5/2 = 35/12 = 2\,11/12$
2d   $1/500 \times 5 = 1/500 \times 5/1 = 5/500 = 1/100$
2e   $8\,3/4 \times 3/120 = 35/4 \times 3/120 = 105/480 = 21/96 = 7/32$

3a   $3/5 \div 4/5 = 3/5 \times 5/4 = 15/20 = 3/4$
3b   $19\,1/4 \div 3 = 77/4 \div 3/1 = 77/4 \times 1/3 = 77/12 = 6\,5/12$
3c   $1/50 \div 1/200 = 1/50 \times 200/1 = 200/50 = 4$
3d   $11 \div 3\,3/4 = 11/1 \div 15/4 = 11/1 \times 4/15 = 44/15 = 2\,14/15$
3e   $1/8 \div 8 = 1/8 \div 8/1 = 1/8 \times 1/8 = 1/64$

4a   $3/8 + 5/16 = 6/16 + 5/16 = 11/16$
4b   $9/13 + 1/3 = 27/39 + 13/39 = 40/39 = 1\,1/39$
4c   $1\,5/8 + 3\,3/4 + 5\,3/10 = 13/8 + 15/4 + 53/10 = 65/40 + 150/40 + 212/40 = 427/40 = 10\,27/40$
4d   $10\,1/2 + 5 + 6\,1/3 = 21/2 + 5/1 + 19/3 = 63/6 + 30/6 + 38/6 = 131/6 = 21\,5/6$
4e   $3\,2/3 + 5\,1/2 + 5/11 = 11/3 + 11/2 + 5/11 = 242/66 + 363/66 + 30/66 = 635/66 = 9\,41/66$

5a   $4/5 - 3/10 = 8/10 - 3/10 = 5/10 = 1/2$
5b   $5\,1/12 - 2/3 = 61/12 - 2/3 = 61/12 - 8/12 = 53/12 = 4\,5/12$
5c   $11\,3/4 - 9\,1/2 = 47/4 - 19/2 = 47/4 - 38/4 = 9/4 = 2\,1/4$
5d   $3/100 - 1/150 = 9/300 - 2/300 = 7/300$
5e   $7\,2/5 - 2/3 = 37/5 - 2/3 = 111/15 - 10/15 = 101/15 = 6\,11/15$

6    $3/4 + 1/2 + 2 + 1\,5/8 = 3/4 + 1/2 + 2/1 + 13/8 = 6/8 + 4/8 + 16/8 + 13/8 = 39/8 = 4\,7/8$ pounds

7    $4\,7/8 - 1\,1/2 = 39/8 - 3/2 = 39/8 - 12/8 = 27/8 = 3\,3/8$ pounds eaten

8    $3/8 + 1\,1/2 + 3/16 + 2 = 3/8 + 3/2 + 3/16 + 2/1 = 6/16 + 24/16 + 3/16 + 32/16 = 65/16 = 4\,1/16$ pounds

9    *Step 1*  $3 \times 1\,1/4 = 3/1 \times 5/4 = 15/4 = 3\,3/4$ pounds used
     *Step 2*  $4\,1/16$ lb $- 3\,3/4$ pounds used $= 65/16 - 1\,5/4 = 65/16 - 60/16 = 5/16$ pounds

10   24 teaspoons $\div 3/4 = 24/1 \div 3/4 = 24/1 \times 4/3 = 96/3 = 32$ doses

11   5 tablets $\times 1/150$ grains $= 5 \times 1/150 = 5/1 \times 1/150 = 5/150 = 1/30$

12   $3/16$ ounce $\div 30$ capsules $= 3/16 \div 30/1 = 3/16 \times 1/30 = 3/480 = 1/160$ ounces

13a  $15 + 1.5 + 0.15 + 150 = 166.65$
13b  $3.25 + 13.091 + 0.18 = 16.521$
13c  $0.38 + 0.097 + 0.0062 = 0.4832$
13d  $22.0008 + 8.022 = 30.0228$

14a $32 - 1.0009 = 30.9991$
14b $2.52 - 0.333 = 2.187$
14c $491.08 - 321.008 = 170.072$
14d $0.0678 - 0.00678 = 0.06102$

15a $23.8 \div 0.294 = 80.952$
15b $0.91 \div 8.27 = 0.11$
15c $341.44 \div 0.37 = 922.81$
15d $68.2 \div 2000 = 0.0341$

16a $0.003 \times 0.09 = 0.00027$
16b $54.5 \times 25.12 = 1369.04$
16c $100.25 \times 100.35 = 10,060.087$
16d $1336 \times 10,000 = 13,360,000$

17a $XXIV \times 3.25 = 24 \times 3.25 = 78$
17b $26.23 \times 6\ 7/12 = 26.23 \times 6.583 = 172.68$
17c $LXVI + 41.9 + 333\ 1/2 = 66 + 41.9 + 333.5 = 441.4$
17d $(cxiiiss)(8\ 3/8) = 113.5 \times 8.375 = 950.56$
17e $LXVII - XLII = 67 - 42 = 25 = XXV$
17f $17.1 \div 4\ 3/8 = 17.1 \div 4.375 = 3.91$
17g $3\ 3/4 \div 3.089 = 3.75 \div 3.089 = 1.214$
17h $5.029 \times 19\ 7/8 = 5.029 \times 19.875 = 99.95$
17i $13\ 1/4 \div 1/50 = 53/4 \div 1/50 = 53/4 \times 50/1 = 2650/4 = 662.5$
$= DCLXIISS$
17j $6.25 \times 5/8 = 6.25 \times 0.625 = 3.91$
17k $1/4 \times ? = 48 \qquad 48 \div 1/4 = ? \qquad 192 = ?$
check answer $1/4 \times 192 = 48$
17l $(0.5 \div 2) \times ? = 2 \qquad (0.25) \times ? = 2 \qquad 2 \div 0.25 = 8$
check answer $(0.25) \times 8 = 2$
17m $(1/12 \div 1/15) \times 30 = ? \qquad (1.25) \times 30 = ? \qquad 37.5 = ?$

NOTE: It is easiest to convert all common fractions to decimal fractions.

18 $96 \div 4\ 4/5 = 96 \div 4.8 = 20$ salads

19 $XXXII \div 8.5 = 32 \div 8.5 = 3.76$ ounces

20 $MDCXXXV \div CIX = 1635 \div 109 = 15$ technicians

21 *Step 1* (Determine how much has been dispensed.)
30 capsules $\times$ 1.25 = 37.50 grams
15 capsules $\times$ 2.75 = 41.25 grams
10 capsules $\times$ 1.5 = 15.00 grams
93.75 grams dispensed

*Step 2* 100 grams − 93.75 grams = 6.25 grams remaining

22 6.25 grams remaining $\div 1\ 3/4 = 6.25 \div 1.75 = 3.57$, but only three capsules can be completely filled.

23 $32.5 + 15\ 3/8 + 75.5 + 118\ 1/8 = 32.5 + 15.375 + 75.5 + 118.125 = 241.5 = CCXLISS$

24 $3/4 \div 0.00055 = 0.75 \div 0.00055 = 1363.63$

25 $\$350 \times 0.001 = \$0.35$

26 $1/8 + 1/4 + 1\ 1/2 = 1\ 7/8. \quad 4 - 1\ 7/8 = 2\ 1/8$

27 $20 \times 5.5 = 110 = CX$

28 $45\ g \div 60,000$ tablets $= 0.00075$ grams per tablet

29 $14 + 4.75 + 3.75 = 22.5$ milliliters (amount used)
$58 - 22.5 = 35.5$ milliliters (amount remaining)

30 $1\ 1/2 \div 12 = 3/2 \div 12/1 = 3/2 \times 1/12 = 3/24 = 1/8$

31 $2\ 2/3 \times 24 = 8/3 \times 24/1 = 192/3 = 64$ ounces

32 $7.5$ milliliters $\times 3 = 22.5$ milliliters per day
$400$ milliliters $\div 22.5$ milliliters/day $= 17.8$ days,
but only 17 full days

33 $1\ 2/3 \times 7 = 5/3 \times 7/1 = 35/3 = 11.67$ ounces in week 1
$11.67 \times 1/2 = 5.83$ ounces in week 2
$11.67 + 5.83 = 17.5$ ounces

34 $220$ microgram/actuation $\times 1/5 = 44$ microgram per actuation strength

35 $16/100 + 28/100 + 25/100 = 69/100$ gram per packet
$69/100 \times 100$ packets $= 6900/100 = 69$ grams per box

## CHAPTER 2

1a 25 kilograms = 25,000 grams
1b 55 grams = 55,000 milligrams
1c 72 milligrams = 72,000 micrograms
1d 105 liters = 105,000 milliliters
1e 48 meters = 4800 centimeters
1f 1257 millimeters = 1.257 meters
1g 387 centimeters = 3870 millimeters
1h 43 millimeters = 4.3 centimeters
1i 982 milligrams = 0.982 gram
1j 3389 milligrams = 0.003389 kilogram
1k 0.0765 milligram = 76.5 micrograms
1l 0.00376 gram = 3760 micrograms
1m 5786 milliliters = 5.786 liters
1n 0.0698 liter = 69.8 milliliters
1o 0.00997 kilogram = 9970 milligrams
1p 8,023,766 grams = 8023.766 kilograms
1q 7569 micrograms = 0.007569 gram
1r 355.56 milliliters = 0.35556 liter
1s 0.0298 meter = 29.8 millimeters
1t 0.002289 milliliter = 0.000002289 liter
1u 0.200897 kilogram = 200,897,000 micrograms

2 635 g + 0.58 kg + 428,970 mg = 635 g + 580 g + 428.97 g
= 1643.97 g

3 1.27 kg $\div$ 429 grapes = 1270 g $\div$ 429 grapes = 2.96 g each

4     454 g ÷ 22,700 mg/pot = 454 g ÷ 22.7 g/pot = 20 pots of coffee

5     1.89 L ÷ 210 mL/glass = 1890 mL ÷ 210 mL = 9 glasses

6     2.6 km × 2 = 5.2 km = 5200 m

7     8 lb × 454 g/lb = 3632 g = 3.632 kg

8     99 bandages × 7.62 cm = 754.38 cm = 7.5438 m

9     378 g + 0.86 kg + 198,000 mg + 38,000,000 mcg
      = 378 g + 860 g + 198 g + 38 g = 1474 g

10    1.5 kg − 1474 g = 1500 g − 1474 g = 26,000 mg needed

11    3.84 L ÷ 120 mL/bottle = 3840 mL ÷ 120 mL = 32 bottles

12    3 kg ÷ 90 g/shaker = 3000 g ÷ 90 = 33.33 shakers
      or 33 "full" shakers

13    2500 capsules × 750 mcg = 1,875,000 mcg = 1875 mg
      = 1.875 grams

14    0.0009 kg ÷ 30 mg/capsule = 900 mg ÷ 30 mg = 30 capsules

15    40 mg tobramycin in 1 mL = 4 mg/0.1 mL = 4000 mcg

16    178 cm = 1780 mm

17a   5 quarts = 5 quarts × 32 ounces/quart = 160 fluid ounces
17b   3 gallons = 3 gallons × 8 pints/gallon = 24 pints
17c   498 pints = 498 pt ÷ 8 pints/gallons = 62.25 gallons
17d   322 fl. ounces = 322 fl. ounces ÷ 32 fl. ounces per quart
      = 10.06 quarts
17e   960 minims = 960 minims ÷ 480 minims per fluid ounce
      = 2 fluid ounces
17f   480 fl. drams = 480 fl. drams ÷ 8 fl. drams per fl. ounce
      = 60 fluid ounces
17g   1/4 gallon = 1/4 gallon × 8 pints/gallon = 2 pints
17h   76 ounces = 76 ounces × 480 grains/ounce = 36,480 grains
17i   64 drams = 64 drams ÷ 8 drams/ounce = 8 ounces

NOTE: It is important to *estimate* when working all problems.
Estimation is essential in understanding whether to multiply
or divide by conversion factors. Try to estimate more if you had
difficulty with the previous questions.

18    2 gallons ÷ 4 fl ounces/bottle = 256 fl ounces ÷ 4 fl ounces
      = 64 bottles

19    *Step 1*  180 gr × 7 days = 1260 grains/week
      *Step 2*  1260 grains ÷ 480 grains/ounce = 2.625 gr

20    1 3/4 ounces ÷ 1 3/4 gr/capsule = 840 gr ÷ 1.75 gr/capsule
      = 480 capsules

21a   168 lb = 168 lb × 16 oz per lb = 2688 oz
21b   137 oz = 137 oz ÷ 16 oz per lb = 8.56 lb
21c   36 oz = 36 oz × 437.5 gr per oz = 15,750 gr
21d   768 gr = 768 gr ÷ 7000 gr per lb = 0.1097 lb
21e   1276 gr = 1276 gr ÷ 437.5 gr per oz = 2.92 oz

22    1 1/8 lb + 15 oz + 3276 gr = 18 oz + 15 oz + 7.49 oz = 40.49 oz

NOTE: Your answers may be a little different than mine based on
the *conversion factors* being used. All of the following problems
can be worked several different ways.

23a   4.5 tsp = 4.5 tsp × 5 mL per tsp = 22.5 mL
23b   325 lb = 325 lb ÷ 2.2 lb per kg = 147.7 kg
23c   3000 gr = 3000 gr ÷ 15.4 gr per gram = 194.81 g
23d   289 kg = 289 kg × 2.2 lb per kg = 635.8 lb
23e   75 mL = 75 mL ÷ 5 mL per tsp = 15 tsp
23f   67 g = 67 g × 15.4 gr per g = 1031.8 g
23g   6.5 lb = 6.5 lb × 16 oz per lb = 104 oz
23h   118 mg = 118 mg ÷ 65 mg per grain = 1.82 gr
23i   727 oz = 727 oz ÷ 16 oz per lb = 45.44 lb
23j   1700 mL = 1700 mL ÷ 480 mL per pint = 3.54 pints
23k   43 gr = 43 gr × 65 mg per gr = 2795 mg
23l   35 tbsp = 35 tbsp × 3 tsp per tbsp = 105 tsp
23m   4.8 pints = 4.8 pints × 480 mL per pint = 2304 mL
23n   3 fl ounces = 3 fl ounces × 6 tsp per fl ounce = 18 tsp
23o   64 fl ounces = 64 fl ounces ÷ 16 fl ounces per pint = 4 pints
23p   111 kg = 111 kg × 2.2 lb per kg = 244.2 lb
23q   485 lb = 485 lb ÷ 2.2 lb per kg = 220.45 kg
23r   4 quarts = 4 quarts × 960 mL per quart = 3840 mL = 3.84 L
23s   15,000 mL = 15,000 mL ÷ 3840 mL per gallon = 3.91 gallons
23t   5 3/4 lb = 5 3/4 lb × 454 g per lb = 2610.5 g
23u   2150 mL = 2150 mL ÷ 15 mL per tbsp = 143.3 tbsp
23v   3 1/2 oz = 3.5 oz × 28.4 g per oz = 99.4 g
23w   35 pints = 35 pints ÷ 8 pints/gallon = 4.375 gallons
23x   5 L = 5000 mL = 5000 mL ÷ 480 mL/pint = 10.42 pints
23y   4000 mL = 4000 mL ÷ 30 mL/fl. oz. = 133.3 fl. oz.
23z   350 tsp = 350 tsp × 5 mL/tsp = 1750 mL = 1.75 L

24a   18 gr + 2600 mg + 1.3 g + 1/4 oz = 18 gr + 40 gr + 20 gr
      + 109.4 gr = 187.4 gr
24b   187.4 gr = 187.4 gr × 65 mg per gr = 12,181 mg
      (or 12.181 g for question 24c)
24c   1/2 oz = 1/2 oz × 28.4 g per oz = 14.2 g in stock
      − 12.181 g dispensed = 2.019 g

25a   1/8 gal + 1/2 qt + 1/2 pt + 5 fl oz + 8 tbsp + 15 tsp
      = 480 mL + 480 mL + 240 mL + 150 mL + 120 mL + 75 mL
      = 1545 mL = 309 tsp
25b   1 gallon − 1545 mL = 3840 mL − 1545 mL
      = 2295 mL remain

26    50 mL + 480 mL + 960 mL + 750 mL = 2240 mL (removed)
      4000 mL − 2240 mL = 1760 mL (remaining in the bag)

27    500 mcg × 21 days = 10,500 mcg = 10.5 mg = 0.0105 g

28    480 mL ÷ 1,000,000 capsules = 0.00048 mL per capsule

29a   2000 g ÷ 40,000 tablets = 0.05 g = 50 mg per tablet
29b   60 tablets × 50 mg = 3000 mg = 3 g

30    15 mL × 4 doses × 7 days = 420 mL (used)
      480 mL − 420 mL = 60 mL (remaining in bottle)
      If each dose is 15 mL, then 60 mL ÷ 15 mL/dose = 4 doses
      remaining in bottle

31a   1 gallon = 128 ounces
      3 quarts = 96 ounces
      7 pints = 112 ounces
      36 bottles = 216 ounces
      552 total ounces × 30 mL/ounce = 16,560 mL
31b   552 ounces ÷ 128 ounces/gallon = 4.31 gallons

32a   66 lb ÷ 2.2 lb/kg = 30 kg
32b   10 mg/kg would be the same as saying 10 mg/2.2 lb

33a   6 pounds × 16 ounces/lb = 96 ounces
      96 ounces + 15 ounces = 111 ounces
33b   111 ounces × 28.4 grams/ounce = 3152 grams = 3.152 kg

NOTE: There are many ways to solve this problem, so if you worked
it differently, that is OK, as long as you got the correct answer.

34a   1/150 gr × 65 mg/gr = 0.43 mg

NOTE: Sometimes you will see 0.4 mg on a bottle of nitroglycerin
1/150 gr because some manufacturers use 60 mg/gr, but it is best
for you to use 65 mg/gr in practice.

34b   0.43 mg/tablet × 25 tablets = 10.75 mg = 0.01075 g

35a   16/100 g + 28/100 g + 25/100 g = 69/100 g per packet
      × 10 packets = 690/100 g total
      690/100 = 6.9 g = 6900 mg
35b   25/100 g phosphorus = 0.25 g
      0.25 g × 100 packets = 25 g = 25,000 mg = 25,000,000 mcg

## CHAPTER 3

1a    4/12 = 1/3 = 0.333 = 1:3
1b    20/210 = 2/21 = 0.095 = 2:21*

*NOTE: This is the improper form for writing ratios. We will discuss
the correct configuration in a future chapter.

1c    38/218 = 19/109 = 0.174 = 19:109*
1d    6/10 = 3/5 = 0.6 = 3:5*
1e    5/1000 = 1/200 = 0.005 = 1:200
1f    44/100 = 22/50 = 11/25 = 0.44 = 11:25*
1g    3/15 = 1/5 = 0.2 = 1:5
1h    30/600 = 3/60 = 1/20 = 0.05 = 1:20
1i    600/2400 = 60/240 = 6/24 = 1/4 = 0.25 = 1:4

2    200 calories/2.1 oz = ?/19 oz        ? = 1809.5 calories

3    1 shampoo/5 mL = ?/750 mL            ? = 150 shampoos

4a   75 sheets/1 week = ?/42 weeks
     ? = 3150 sheets of paper per year
4b   75 sheets/1 student = ?/26 students
     ? = 1950 sheets of paper per week

5    2.92 mg sodium/1 fl oz = ?/12 fl oz
     ? = 35.04 mg = 0.03504 g

6    1500 rumples/$1 = 480,000 rumples/?
     ? = $320

7    12 diapers/1 day = ?/14 days         ? = 168 diapers (whew!)

8    18 miles/8 pints (gallon) = 698 miles/?
     ? = 310.22 pints

9    1.2 mg/1 fl oz = ?/8 fl oz
     ? = 9.6 mg = 9600 mcg

10   1 Rx/135 seconds = ?/3600 seconds (hour)
     ? = 26.7 prescriptions per hour

11   5 mg diazepam/1 tab = ?/500,000 tabs
     ? = 2,500,000 mg = 2.5 kg

12   25 mg expect./15 mL (tbsp) = ?/960 mL (quart)
     ? = 1600 mg expectorant per quart

13   182 lb sulfur/$2134 = 3 lb/?         ? = $35.18

14   20 mg antiflatulent/0.3 mL = ?/30 mL
     ? = 2000 mg = 2 g antiflatulent

15   5 gr ASA/1 tablet = ?/250 tablets
     ? = 1250 gr = 81.17 g ASA

16   10 g ZnO/100 g oint. = 170.25 g ZnO/?
     ? = 1,702.5 g of ointment
     (3/8 pound = 3/8 × 454 g = 170.25 g)

17   1 kg/2.2 lb = ?/186 lb               ? = 84.55 kg

18   0.25 mg alpr./1 tab = ?/100 tabs     ? = 25 mg = 0.385 gr

19   960 mg med/480 mL (pint) = ?/10 mL (2 tsp)
     ? = 20 mg = 0.02 g

20   NOTE: 1/150 gr = 0.00667 gr
     0.00667 gr/1 tablet = ?/30 tablets   ? = 0.2 gr = 13 mg

21   1.4 mL/1 minute = ?/1440 minutes (1 day)
     ? = 2016 mL = 2.016 L

22 0.75 mg (750 mcg)/1 vial = 15 mg/?     ? = 20 vials

23 $32/3840 mL (gal) = ?/1000 mL     ? = $8.33

24 2270 g sugar/3000 mL = ?/5 mL     ? = 3.78 g sugar

25 130 mg (2 gr)/90 capsules = ?/1 capsule
? = 1.444 mg or 1444 mcg

26 5 mL × 3 doses/day × 7 days = 105 mL per week
$128.31/480 mL = ?/105 mL     ? = $28.07

27 1 gr/65 mg = 0.01 gr/?     ? = 0.65 mg
1 tablet/0.65 mg = 60 tablets/?     ? = 39 mg

28 16 oz/$83.76 = 3 oz/?     ? = $15.71

29 1 fl oz/50 mg = 0.5 fl oz/?     ? = 25 mg
65 mg/1 gr = 25 mg/?     ? = 0.38 gr

30 65 mg/1 gr = ?/ 3/4 gr     ? = 48.75 mg
2 mg/1 tablet = 48.75 mg/?     ? = 24.375 tablets

31 20 mg/1 tablet = 500 mg/?     ? = 25 tablets

32 125 mg/5 mL = 50 mg/?     ? = 2 mL

33 200 mL/1 hr = ?/24 hr     ? = 4800 mL = 4.8 L
1 bag/1 L = ?/4.8 L     ? = 4.8 bags
(so you would need five 1–liter bags)

34 80 mg/2 mL = 10 mg/?     ? = 0.25 mL

35 15 drops/1 mL = ?/500 mL     ? = 7500 drops

36a 16:69 or 1:4.3
36b 28:25 potassium to phosphorus

37a 7.5/650 = 1/?
? = 86.7 so the correct ratio is 1:86.7
37b 7.5 mg/1 tab = ?/0.5 tab     ? = 3.75 mg
3.75 mg = 0.00375 g

38a 1 tab/0.1 mg = 14 tab/?     ? = 1.4 mg = 1400 mcg
38b 1 tab/1 gr = 100 tab/?     ? = 100 gr
1 gr/65 mg = 100 gr/?     ? = 6500 mg = 6.5 g

39a 1 tab/25 mg = 90 tab/?     ? = 2250 mg = 2.25 g
39b 1 tab/100 mg = 0.5 tab/?     ? = 50 mg
50 mg/day × 7 days = 350 mg = 350,000 mcg

40a 500 mg/1000 g = ?/260 g     ? = 130 mg per day
130 mg/day × 30 days = 3900 mg = 3.9 g
40b 500 mg/kg/day is the same as saying 500 mg/2.2 lb/day
500 mg/2.2 lb = ?/1 lb     ? = 227 mg per lb

# CHAPTER 4

1a Put (instill) 3 drops in right eye every 6 hours as needed for pain.
1b One tablet under the tongue (sublingually) as needed for shortness of breath.
1c Take 2 capsules by mouth after meals and at bedtime.
1d Inject 5 units of Humulin® insulin subcutaneously now.
1e Give 1 gram of Ancef® by intravenous piggyback every 6 hours.
1f Take 10 mg of Inderal® by mouth four times a day.
1g Take 1 Dalmane® 15-mg capsule by mouth at bedtime.
1h Take 2 puffs of Atrovent® inhaler 4 times a day as directed.
1i Instill 2 drops of Cortisporin Otic® in both ears three times a day.
1j Take 1 teaspoonful of Cefzil® twice a day for 10 days.
1k Take 2 Persantine® 50-mg tablets 4 times a day, 30 minutes before meals.

2 Patient name, drug name, dose, route, dosage regimen, date (and time), and signature

3 1 capsule × 4 doses × 10 days = 40 capsules

4 Change 0.03 g to 30,000 mcg
200 mcg/1 dose = 30,000 mcg/?     ? = 150 doses

5 2 mg × 3 times a day × 30 days = 180 mg = 0.18 gram

6 4 fl oz = 120 mL = 24 tsp
24 tsp/6 days = ?/1 day     ? = 4 tsp/day

NOTE: It is OK to work problem 6 and all the remaining problems any way you prefer as long as you understand what you are doing and get the correct answers. You might have solved this last problem as:
120 mL/6 days = ?/1 day
? = 20 mL per day or 4 teaspoonfuls

NOTE: Beginning with the next question, I will be converting units in this answer key without further explanation. I believe you have advanced enough to recognize when conversions have been made. In Question 7, there are four different units: milligrams, grams, fluid ounces, and tablespoons. I converted grams to milligrams because the answer is asked for in milligrams. I converted the fluid ounces to tablespoons because it was a lot easier for me. Good luck, and hang in there!

7 360 mg/12 tbsp = ?/1 tbsp
? = 30 mg per tablespoonful

8 50 mcg/1 mL = 500 mcg/?     ? = 10 mL

9 1 inhal./50 mcg = 200 inhal./?     ? = 10,000 mcg = 10 mg

10 5 mL × 3 × 10 = 150 mL

11 200 mcg/1 mL = 125 mcg/?     ? = 0.625 mL

12  120 mL/1 day = 960 mL/?        ? = 8 days

13  50 mg/5 mL = ?/120 mL          ? = 1200 mg

14  50 u/1 mL = ?/20 mL
    ? = 1000 u/hr × 24 hours = 24,000 units per day

15  (10 u × 4 = 40 u/day)
    (100 u/mL = ?/10 mL, then ? = 1000 units per vial)
    40 units/1 day = 1000 units/?        ? = 25 days

16  3 mg/2.2 lb = ?/36 lb          ? = 49.1 mg
    (Did you catch my shortcut?)

17  30 mg/5 mL = 49.1 mg/?         ? = 8.183 mL = 8.2 mL

18  (25 mg/2.2 lb = ?/220 lb       ? = 2500 mg/day × 7 days
    = 17,500 mg per week)
    500 mg/1 capsule = 17,500 mg/?   ? = 35 capsules

19  325 mg/1 tablet = ?/42 tablets   ? = 13,650 mg

20  13,650 mg/20 kg = ?/1 kg
    ? = 682.5 mg (i.e., 682.5 mg/kg)

21  2 puffs × 6 × 42 days = 504 puffs for the vacation
    200 puffs/1 canister = 504 puffs/?
    ? = 2.52 canisters (take 3 on trip)

22  2 mg/1 lb = ?/8.8 lb
    ? = 17.6 mg/day × 5 days = 88 mg total

23  10 mL × 3 × 3 days = 90 mL, *then* 5 mL × 3 × 4 days = 60 mL
    60 mL + 90 mL = 150 mL total
    150 mL/30 mL per fl. oz. = 5 fl. oz.

24  0.4 mg alkaloid/15 mL = ?/1000 mL    ? = 26.67 mg of alkaloid

25  $78.50/960 mL = ?/15 mL        ? = $1.23

26  Use the nomogram for children to get a BSA of 0.75 m²
    for this patient. 0.8 mg/1 m² = ?/0.75 m²
    ? = 0.6 mg = 600 mcg

27  1 kg/2.2 lb = ?/121 lb         ? = 55 kg (patient's weight)
    12 mcg/1 kg = ?/55 kg          ? = 660 mcg = 0.66 mg

28  21 days × 0.66 mg/day = 13.86 mg over 3 weeks
    13.86 mg/$285 = 1 mg/?         ? = $20.56

29  1 kg/2.2 lb = ?/6.6 lb         ? = 3 kg
    2.5 mg/1 kg = ?/3 kg
    ? = 7.5 mg q.12 hr = 15 mg daily

30  1 hr/60 min = 6 hr/?           ? = 360 minutes
    750 mL/360 min = ?/1 min       ? = 2.083 mL per minute

31  0.1 mg = 100 mcg               100 mcg/1 mL = 85 mcg/?
    ? = 0.85 mL

32  25 mg/2 mL = 15 mg/?           ? = 1.2 mL

33  Use adult nomogram to get a BSA of 2.06 m² for this patient.
    20 mg/1 m² = ?/2.06 m²         ? = 41.2 mg daily
    41.2 mg/1 day = ?/7 days       ? = 288.4 mg per week

34  50 mg/1 mL = 20 mg/?           ? = 0.4 mL

35  1 gr/65 mg = 10 gr/?           ? = 650 mg
    160 mg/1.6 mL = 650 mg/?       ? = 6.5 mL

36a 100 units/1 mL = ?/10 mL       ? = 1000 units per vial
    25 units/1 day = 1000 units/?  ? = 40 days

36b Assume that 4 months is approximately 120 days.
    30 units/1 day = ?/120 days    ? = 3600 units
    1000 units/1 vial = 3600 units/?
    ? = 3.6 vials so the patient needs 4 vials

37a 0.025 mg/1 tab = ?/8 tabs      ? = 0.2 mg = 0.0002 g
37b 0.4 mg/2.2 lb = ?/3.5 lb       ? = 0.636 mg = 636 mcg

38a 5 mg/2.2 lb = ?/128 lb         ? = 291 mg
38b 100 mg/1 vial = 291 mg/?
    ? = 2.91 vials so you would need 3 vials

39a 160 mcg/1 inhalation = ?/120 inhalations
    ? = 19,200 mcg = 19.2 mg
39b 0.009 mg = 9 mcg, and a canister contains 120 inhalations
    4.5 mcg/1 inhalation = 9 mcg/?   ? = 2 inhalations daily
    2 inhalations/1 day = 120 inhalations/?
    ? = 60 days

40a 100 units/1 mL = 12 units/?    ? = 0.12 mL
40b 70%

NOTE: It doesn't matter what volume you give; the answer will still
be 70%.

# CHAPTER 5

1a  a.a. means "of each"
1b  ad means "add *up to*"
1c  q.s. means "add a sufficient quantity *to make*"
1d  D.T.D. means "give of such doses"
1e  M. means "mix"
1f  ft. means "make"

2   325 mg aceta./1 tab = ?/5000 tabs
    ? = 1,625,000 mg = 1625 g

3a  30 mg pseudoephedrine × 100 = 3000 mg = 3 grams
3b  2 mg brompheniramine × 100 = 200 mg = 0.2 gram
3c  200 mg ibuprofen × 100 = 20,000 mg = 20 grams

4  12.5 mg/5 mL = ?/480 mL        ? = 1200 mg = 1.2 g

5  500 mg/1 tablet = ?/150 tablets
   ? = 75,000 mg or 75 grams per bottle
   75 g/1 bottle = ?/10,000 bottles     ? = 750,000 g = 750 kg

6a  NOTE: The total formula weight is 10 + 2 + 88 = 100 g.
    10 g pre.sul./100 g = ?/2000 g
    ? = 200 g of precipitated sulfur
6b  2 g sal. ac./100 g = ?/2000 g
    ? = 40 g of salicylic acid
6c  88 g hydr. ung./100 g = ?/2000 g
    ? = 1760 g of hydrophilic oint.

NOTE: The easiest way to answer 6c would be to create a factor, 2000/100 = 20, and multiply everything by that factor. To check your answer, *add* all three components together; they should total 2000 g or 2 kg.

7a  10 g pre. sul./100 g = ?/60 g
    ? = 6 g of precipitated sulfur
7b  2 g sal. ac/100 g = ?/60 g
    ? = 1.2 g of salicylic acid
7c  88 g hydr. ung./100 g = ?/60 g
    ? = 52.8 g of hydrophilic oint.

NOTE: An easier solution to 7c is to multiply each component by the factor 0.6, i.e., 60/100. Check your answer by adding all the components together: 6 + 1.2 + 52.8 = 60 g.

NOTE: Question 8a can be worked by the ratio and proportion process, but let's take the shortcut and create a factor to multiply by each component. The factor is 45/120 = 0.375.

8a  Camphor = 0.375 × 0.3 g = 0.1125 g camphor
8b  Menthol = 0.375 × 2 g = 0.75 g menthol
8c  Talc = 0.375 × 90 g = 33.75 g talc
8d  Zinc oxide (If you multiplied 120 × 0.375, you *killed* the patient! Do not forget, q.s. to 120 g means you add up the other components and subtract them from 120 g to find out how much zinc oxide is needed. In this case, 0.3 + 2 + 90 = 92.3 g, then 120 − 92.3 = 27.7 g of zinc oxide in the original formula. Now multiply this amount by the factor of 0.375.)
    zinc oxide = 0.375 × 27.7 g = 10.39 g zinc oxide
    Now add them together to see if you get 45 g as a final answer: 0.1125 + 0.75 + 33.75 + 10.39 = 45 g

9a  0.3 g camphor/120 g = ?/454 g     ? = 1.135 g camphor
9b  2 g menthol/120 g = ?/454 g       ? = 7.57 g menthol
9c  90 g talc/120 g = ?/454 g         ? = 340.5 g talc
9d  27.7 g zinc oxide/120 g = ?/454 g ? = 104.8 g zinc oxide

NOTE: The factor for problem 9d is 454/120 = 3.783, and all four quantities add up to 454 g.

10  90 mL glycerin/1000 mL = ?/480 mL
    ? = 43.2 mL glycerin to make a pint of the syrup

11  70 mL ipecac/1000 mL = ?/3840 mL
    ? = 268.8 mL of ipecac fl. extract/gal

12a  75 mcg/1 capsule = ?/30 capsules
     ? = 2250 mcg = 2.2 mg reserpine
12b  20 mg furosemide/1 cap = ?/30 caps
     ? = 600 mg = 0.6 g furosemide
12c  15 mg + 0.075 mg + 20 mg = 35.075 mg per capsule
12d  35.075 mg/1 capsule = ?/30 capsules
     ? = 1052.25 mg = 1.052 grams
12e  15 mg hydralazine/30 caps = ?/1 cap
     ? = 0.5 mg = 500 mcg hydralazine/cap

13a  2100 mg/1000 mL = ?/240 mL       ? = 504 mg
13b  100 gr = 6500 mg = 6.5 g
     40 g/1000 mL = 6.5 g/?           ? = 162.5 mL

14a  36 capsules × 30 mg Pb/capsule = 1080 mg Pb needed
     60 mg Pb/1 tablet = 1080 mg Pb/?   ? = 18 tablets
14b  0.6 g × 36 capsules = 21.6 g = 21,600 mg
     1 gr/65 mg = ?/21,600 mg          ? = 332.3 grains

15a  250 g/1000 tablets = ?/40,000 tablets
     ? = 10,000 g = 10 kg
15b  2 pounds = 908 grams (454 × 2)
     150 g/1000 tablets = 908 g/?      ? = 6053 tablets

16a  5 gr = 325 mg (5 × 65 mg)        325 mg/1 cap = ?/64 caps
     ? = 20,800 mg = 20.8 g = 0.0208 kg
16b  1/2 gr/1 cap = ?/64 caps          ? = 32 grains total
     1 gr/65 mg = 32 gr/?              ? = 2080 mg = 2.08 g
     30 g/$8.50 = 2.08 g/?            ? = $0.59

17a  2.5 mg/1 capsule = ?/24 capsules   ? = 60 mg
     5 mg/1 tablet = 60 mg/?            ? = 12 tablets needed
17b  10 gr = 650 mg (10 × 65 mg)
     650 mg + 2.5 mg = 652.5 mg per capsule
     652.5 mg/1 capsule = ?/24 capsules
     ? = 15,660 mg = 15.66 g

18a  Total weight of electrolytes per 3.2-g packet is 0.69 g.
     3.2 − 0.69 = 2.51 g = 2510 mg inert filler
18b  The ratio strength doesn't change according to the number of packets.
     0.28 g per 3.2 g packet            0.28:3.2
     0.28/3.2 = 1/?
     ? = 11.4 so the ratio strength is 1:11.4
18c  0.25 g/1 packet = ?/100 packets    ? = 25 g per box
     25 g/1 box = ?/10,000 boxes        ? = 250,000 g = 250 kg
18d  0.16 g/1 packet = ?/30 packets     ? = 4.8 g = 4800 mg

19a  0.5 mg/1 vial = ?/30 vials         ? = 15 mg
19b  3 mg/1 vial = ?/0.5 vial           ? = 1.5 mg = 1500 mcg
19c  0.5 mg/3 mL is the same as 0.0005 g/3 mL
     0.0005 g/3 mL = 0.00017 = 0.017%

20a 230 mcg + 21 mcg = 251 mcg active drug      12,000 mg total weight in a canister
251 mcg × 120 inhalations = 30,120 mcg
= 30.12 mg of active drug in a canister
12,000 mg − 30.12 mg = 11,970 mg inert ingredients per canister

20b 21 mcg/inhalation = ?/120 inhalations
? = 2520 mcg = 2.52 mg
2.52 mg/1 canister = ?/100 canisters
? = 252 mg = 0.252 g = 0.000252 kg

20c If there are 120 actuations in a normal canister, then half a canister would be 60 actuations.
230 mcg/1 actuation = ?/60 actuations
? = 13,800 mcg = 13.8 mg = 0.0138 g

# CHAPTER 6

1a 125 mg/5 mL = ?/200 mL
? = 5000 mg ampicillin in bottle

1b 200 mL final volume − 158 mL of diluent
= 42 mL dry powder volume

1c 178 mL diluent + 42 mL powder volume = 220 mL

1d 5000 mg/220 mL = ?/10 mL      ? = 227.3 mg ampicillin

1e 5000 mg/220 mL = 250 mg/?      ? = 11 mL

2a 125 mg/5 mL = ?/150 mL
? = 3750 mg cefaclor per bottle

2b 150 mL final volume − 111 mL diluent = 39 mL dry volume

2c 100 mg/5 mL = 3750 mg/?      ? = 187.5 mL
187.5 mL − 150 mL = 37.5 additional mL of water

2d 78 mL diluent + 39 mL dry volume = 117 mL final volume
3750 mg/117 mL = ?/5 mL      ? = 160.3 mg per 5 mL

2e 3750 mg/117 mL = 100 mg/?      ? = 3.12 mL

3a 100 mg/1 mL = 300 mg/?      ? = 3 mL

3b 100 mg/1 mL = ?/10 mL
? = 1000 mg = 1 g/vial

3c 250 mg × 4 × 10 days = 10,000 mg total
1000 mg/1 vial = 10,000 mg/?      ? = 10 vials

3d 10 mL final volume − 7.8 mL diluent = 2.2 mL dry volume

3e 9.8 mL diluent + 2.2 mL dry volume = 12 mL final volume
1000 mg/12 mL = 250 mg/?      ? = 3 mL

4a 500,000 u/1 mL = 2,500,000 u/?      ? = 5 mL

4b 500,000 u/1 mL = 10,000,000 u/?      ? = 20 mL

4c 20 mL final volume − 7 mL powder volume = 13 mL of diluent

4d 20 mL diluent + 7 mL powder volume = 27 mL final volume
10,000,000 u/27 mL = ?/1 mL      ? = 370, 370 units/mL

4e 10,000,000 u/27 mL = 2,500,000 u/?      ? = 6.75 mL

5a 15 mL (final volume) − 9 mL (diluent) = 6 mL (dry powder volume)

5b 200 mg/5 mL = ?/15 mL      ? = 600 mg

5c 100 mg daily × 5 days = 500 mg total
600 mg/15 mL = 500 mg/?      ? = 12.5 mL

5d 600 mg/15 mL = ?/3.75 mL      ? = 150 mg = 0.15 g

5e 19 mL (diluent) + 6 mL (dry powder volume) = 25 mL (final volume)

5f There are 600 mg of azithromycin in this bottle no matter how much diluent is added. 600 mg/25 mL = 100 mg/?
? = 4.17 mL = 4.2 mL

6a 250 mg/1 mL = 1000 mg/?      ? = 4 mL (final volume)

6b 4 mL (total volume) − 3.6 mL (diluent) = 0.4 mL (dry powder volume)

6c 1000 mg/4 mL = 350 mg/?      ? = 1.4 mL, or you can say 250 mg/1 mL = 350 mg/?
? = 1.4 mL

6d 2.6 mL (diluent) + 0.4 mL (dry powder volume) = 3 mL (final volume). The vial contains 1000 mg of antibiotic; this amount is not affected by the diluent. 1000 mg/3 mL = 350 mg/?
? = 1.05 mL

7a 57 mg/5 mL = ?/75 mL      ? = 855 mg = 0.855 g

7b 400 mg/5 mL = ?/15 mL      ? = 1200 mg = 1.2 g

7c 75 mL (final volume) − 67 mL (water) = 8 mL

7d 40 mg/2.2 lb = ?/94 lb
? = 1709 mg/day (divided into 3 doses)
1709/3 doses = 570 mg/dose
400 mg/5 mL = 570 mg/?
? = 7.125 mL dose, so you would likely recommend 7 mL.

7e In a correctly compounded suspension, there are 57 mg of clavulanic acid per 5 mL.
57 mg/5 mL = ?/75 mL      ? = 855 mg clavulanic acid per bottle
This quantity does not change with the volume of water added in reconstituting the suspension.
57 mL (water) + 8 mL (dry powder volume)
= 65 mL (final solution)
855 mg/65 mL = ?/5 mL
? = 65.8 mg per teaspoonful dose

7f In a correctly compounded suspension, there are 400 mg amoxicillin/5 mL.
400 mg/5 mL = ?/75 mL
? = 6000 mg in the bottle      That does not change.
6000 mg/65 mL = ?/15 mL      ? = 1385 mg in 15 mL

7g Simply add 10 additional milliliters of water.

8a The vial contains 2 g = 2000 mg aztreonam, and this amount doesn't change with the volume of diluent.

8b 2 g:10 mL or 1:5

8c 3 mL diluent/1 g aztreonam
A minimum of 3 mL of diluent is needed.

# CHAPTER 7

1a 1200 mL/8 hr = ?/1 hr      ? = 150 mL/hr

1b 1200 mL/480 min = ?/5 min      ? = 12.5 mL per 5 min

1c 15 gtt/1 mL = ?/1200 mL      ? = 18,000 gtt

1d 18,000 gtt/480 min = ?/1 min      ? = 37.5 gtt/min

1e 2000 mg/8 hr = ?/1 hr      ? = 250 mg/h

NOTE: You probably worked some of these problems differently, and that is cool as long as your answers were correct. I can think of numerous ways to work these problems.

2a    500 mL/480 min = ?/1 min          ? = 1.042 mL per min
2b    60 gtt/mL = ?/1.042 mL            ? = 62.5 = 63 drops per min
2c    2 mL/1 min = 500 mL/?             ? = 250 min
2d    60 gtt/1 mL = ?/2 mL              ? = 120 drops per min
2e    2000 mcg/500 mL = ?/1 mL          ? = 4 mcg per mL

3a    15 gtt/mL = 40 gtt/?              ? = 2.67 mL per min
3b    2.67 mL/1 min = ?/1440 min        ? = 3845 mL per day
3c    Looks like 3.845 liters, or 4 liter bags
3d    2.67 mL/1 min = ?/60 min          ? = 160 mL per hour
      1000 mg drug/1000 mL = ?/160 mL   ? = 160 mg per hour
3e    160 mg/60 min = ?/1 min
      ? = 2.67 mg = 2670 mcg per min

4a    1000 mL/6 hr = ?/1 hr             ? = 166.7 mL/hr
4b    2,000,000 u/6 hr = ?/1 hr         ? = 333,333 units per hour
4c    2,000,000 u/360 min = ?/1 min     ? = 5556 units per min
4d    1000 mL/360 min = ?/1 min         ? = 2.78 mL/min
4e    1000 mL/6 hr = ?/1 hr             ? = 166.7 mL/hr
      12 gtt/1 mL = ?/166.7 mL          ? = 2000 drops per hour
4f    12 gtt/1 mL = ?/1000 mL           ? = 12,000 total drops
      2,000,000 u/12,000 gtt = ?/1 gtt  ? = 166.7 units per drop

5a    100 mg/1 hr = ?/24 hr             ? = 2400 mg = 2.4 g
5b    2400 mg/2000 mL = 100 mg/?        ? = 83.3 ml/h
5c    2000 mL/1440 min = ?/1 min        ? = 1.39 ml/min
5d    15 gtt/1 mL = ?/1.39 mL
      ? = 20.85 = 21 drops per min
5e    2000 mL/24 hr = ?/5 hr            ? = 416.7 mL in 5 hours
5f    100 mg/1 hr = ?/3.5 hr            ? = 350 mg in 3.5 hours

6a    1000 mL/12 hr = ?/3.75 hr         ? = 312.5 mL
6b    1000 mL/720 min = ?/1 min         ? = 1.39 mL per min
      15 gtt/1 mL = ?/1.39 mL           ? = 20.85 = 21 gtt/min

7a    60 gtt/1 mL = 50 gtt/?            ? = 0.833 mL/min
      0.833 mL/1 min = 50 mL/?          ? = 60 min
      (alternate method)
      60 gtt/1 mL = ?/50 mL             ? = 3000 gtt total
      50 gtt/1 min = 3000 gtt/?         ? = 60 min
7b    50 mL/60 min = ?/10 min           ? = 8.33 mL = 0.0083 L

8a    1000 mL/480 min = ?/1 min         ? = 2.08 mL/min
      12 gtt/1 mL = ?/2.08 mL           ? = 25 gtt/min
8b    1000 mL/8 hr = ?/1 hr             ? = 125 mL
      (Did you make this harder than it was?)

9a    80 mL/1 hr = 1000 mL/?            ? = 12.5 hr
9b    10 am + 12.5 hr = 10:30 pm

10a   2500 units/500 mL = ?/10 mL       ? = 50 units
10b   10 mL/60 min = ?/1 min            ? = 0.167 mL/min
      12 gtt/1 mL = ?/0.167 mL          ? = 2 gtt/min

11a   80 mg + 16mg = 96 mg per mL, so 480 mg in 5 mL
11b   125 mL + 5 mL = 130 mL (final volume)        80 mg/mL × 5 mL
      = 400 mg sulfamethoxazole
      400 mg/130 mL = ?/50 mL           ? = 154 mg
11c   130 mL/90 min = ?/1 min           ? = 1.44 mL/min
11d   16 mg/1 mL = ?/5mL                ? = 80 mg per vial
      80 mg/90 min = 40 mg/?            ? = 45 min
11e   400 mg/90 min = ?/38 min          ? = 169 mg

12a   1 vial/5,000,000 units = ?/15,000,000 units
      ? = 3 vials needed per day
      3 vials/1 day = ?/14 days         ? = 42 vials
12b   15,000,000 units/24 hr = ?/8 hr
      ? = 5,000,000 units
12c   2000 mL/1440 min = ?/1 min        ? = 1.39 mL per min
12d   15,000,000/2000 mL = ?/100mL      ? = 750,000 units
12e   15,000,000 units/2000 mL = 1,000,000 units/?
      ? = 133 mL
      16 gtt/1 mL = ?/133 mL            ? = 2128 gtt

# CHAPTER 8

1a    18.75%    3/16      0.1875    3:16*
      *(incorrectly written; to be discussed later)
1b    18.18%    2/11      0.1818    2:11*
1c    18%       18/100    0.18      18:100* (should be reduced)
1d    3.5%      3.5/100   0.035     3.5:100*
1e    61%       61/100    0.61      61:100*
1f    8%        8/100     0.08      8:100* (should be reduced)
1g    0.8%      1/125     0.008     1:125 (This is the only correctly
      written ratio.)
1h    8.75%     35/400    0.0875    35:400* (should be reduced)

2a    12 fl oz/128 fl oz (gallon) = ?/100 fl oz
      ? = 9.375/100 = 9.375%
2b    1 pint/8 pints (gallon) = ?/100 pints   ? = 12.5/100 = 12.5%
2c    480 mL + 960 mL + 180 mL + 180 mL + 120 mL = 1920 mL
      (You could also work in ounces.)
      1920 mL/3840 mL (gallon) = ?/100 mL   ? = 50/100 = 50%
2d    100% − 50% = 50% (left over for the rest of my herd!)

I will give you all future answers in percentages. I assume you
understand that they mean ?/100.

3a    5 trout/30 trout = ?/100 trout       ? = 16.7%
3b    20 trout/30 trout = ?/100 trout      ? = 66.7%
3c    2.2 lb/1 kg = 22.5 lb/?              ? = 10.23 kg
3d    950 g/10,230 g = ?/100 g             ? = 9.29%
3e    18 escaped/48 total (30 + 18) = ?/100 trout
      ? = 37.5% escaped

4     25 g fat/100 g steak = ?/454 g steak    ? = 113.5 g of fat (yuck!)

5     4 oz fat/14 oz chops = ?/100 oz chops    ? = 28.6% fat (yuckier!)

6     21 miles/26.2 miles = ?/100 miles    ? = 80.2%

7a  28 g protein/448 g beans = ?/100 g beans
    ? = 6.25% protein
7b  2 g fat/100 g beans = ?/448 g beans   ? = 8.96 g fat
7c  448 g total − 68 g carbohydrate = 380 g are not carbohydrate;
    380 g *non*-carbs/448 g beans = ?/100 g beans
    ? = 84.8% *non*-carbohydrate

8a  12 g coal tar/150 g ung = ?/100 g ung   ? = 8% coal tar
8b  Answer 8% (This is a biggie! If the final product is 8%, then
    1 g, 1 kg, 1 oz, 1 lb, 1 ton, etc., of the product is still 8%. Please
    do not forget this.) To prove my point, let's check our answer.
    12,000 mg C.T./150,000 mg ung = ?/100 mg
    ? = 8 mg or (8 mg/100 mg = 0.08 = 8%)

9a  2 mg drug/1 g powder = ?/ 120 g powder
    ? = 240 mg drug in 120 g
9b  2 mg drug/1000 mg powder = ?/100 mg powder
    ? = 0.2% drug in powder

10a 3 g hydrocortisone/100 g cream = ?/454 g cream
    ? = 13.62 g hydrocortisone

NOTE: To check your answer, take the amount of hydrocortisone
and divide it by the total weight of the product.
*Check*: 13.62/454 = 0.03 = 3%

10b 3 g hydrocortisone/100 g cream = ?/1 g cream
    ? = 0.03 g = 30 mg

11a 5 g fluorouracil/100 g cream = ?/25 g cream
    ? = 1.25 g = 1250 mg
11b 5% means you have 1.25 g in the 25 g of cream. If you add
    2 more grams of fluorouracil, you will now have 3.25 g of
    fluorouracil (1.25 + 2 = 3.25), but you must also remember to
    increase the *final* or *total* weight of the cream by 2 g, giving a
    final weight of 27 g (25 + 2 = 27). Now solve the question.
    3.25 g fluorouracil/27 g cream = ?/100 g cream ? = 12.04%

12a 1.5 g hydrocortisone/60 g cream = ?/100 g cream
    ? = 2.5%
12b 60 g total − 2 g hydro and Vio® (1.5 + 0.5 = 2)
    = 58 grams of cream base
12c 1 oz (weight)/28.4 grams = 10 oz/?    ? = 284 g of product
    0.5 g Vioform/60 g product = ?/284 g product
    ? = 2.37 g Vioform powder

13a 200 mg aminophylline/1 suppos. = ?/60 suppos.
    ? = 12,000 mg = 12 g
13b 60 mg + 200 mg + 1800 mg = 2060 mg (weight of 1 suppository)
    = 2.06 grams
    2.06 g/1 suppos. = ?/60 suppos.       ? = 123.6 g
13c As mentioned in question 8b, whatever the percent strength
    is for 1 suppository, it will be the same for 60 suppositories.
    The total weight for 1 suppository is 2060 mg. 60 mg phen/
    2060 mg total wgt. = ?/100 mg wgt.   ? = 2.91% phenobarbital

14a 1 g benzocaine/1000 g product = ?/120 g product
    ? = 0.12 g = 120 mg
14b 10 g pre. sul./100 g product = ?/1000 g product
    ? = 100 g precipitated sulfur
    (*Check*: 100 g sulfur/1000 g product = 0.1 = 10%)

15a Total parts = 14 (2 + 5 + 7 = 14) Now you decide what a part
    is. I picked *grams*. 7 g Ca. carb/14 g powder = ?/908 g powder
    (2 lb)     ? = 454 g calcium carb.
15b 5 parts/14 parts = ?/100 parts       ? = 35.7% sodium
    bicarb.
15c 2 parts magnesium oxide to 14 total parts → 2:14, reduced to 1:7

16a 0.35 mL mint/100 mL m−wash = ?/960 mL m−wash
    ? = 3.36 mL mint flavoring
16b I hope you did not miss this! It is still 0.35% mint flavoring.

17a 16 mL resorcinol/180 mL lotion = ?/100 mL lotion
    ? = 8.89% resorcinol
17b 16 mL resorcinol/180 mL lotion = ?/5000 mL lotion
    ? = 444.4 mL resorcinol

18a 6 mL methyl/100 mL lotion = 480 methyl/?
    ? = 8000 mL = 2.083 gal.
18b 6 mL methyl/100 mL lotion = ?/480 mL lotion
    ? = 28.8 mL methyl sal.
    *Check*: 28.8 mL methyl sal./480 mL lotion = 0.06 = 6%

19  5 mL oil/100 mL *spirits* = 15 mL oil/?
    ? = 300 mL *spirits*

20  1 mL oil/15 mL *spirits* = 240 mL oil/?
    ? = 3600 mL *spirits*

21a 0.9 g NaCl/100 mL sol. = ?/1000 mL sol.
    ? = 9 g sodium chloride
21b 200 mL/1 hr = ?/3 hr              ? = 600 mL
    0.9 g NaCl/100 mL = ?/600 mL      ? = 5.4 g NaCl

22a 37.5 g Na bicarb/500 mL = ?/100 mL
    ? = 7.5% sodium bicarbonate
22b 37.5 g Na bicarb/500 mL = ?/100 mL
    ? = 7.5 g = 7500 mg sodium bicarbonate

NOTE: You could also use your answer from 22a and say that
100 mL × 7.5% = 7.5 g.

22c Please tell me you got this right this time! The percent strength
    is 7.5% no matter what the volume is.

23a 85 g iodine/3840 mL = ?/100 mL      ? = 2.21%
23b 3 g iodine/100 mL tincture = 85 g iodine/?
    ? = 2833 mL 3% tincture
23c 1 g iodine/100 mL tincture = 85 g iodine/?
    ? = 8500 mL 1:100 tincture

24a　25 mg adenosine/1 mL = ?/10 mL　　　? = 250 mg = 0.25 g
24b　25 mg/1 mL = ?/100 mL
　　　? = 2500 mg/100 mL = 2.5 g/100 mL = 2.5%
24c　25 mg adenosine/1 mL = 35 mg adenosine/?
　　　? = 1.4 mL

25a　0.5 g pilocarpine/100 mL sol. = ?/15 mL
　　　? = 0.075 g = 75 mg
25b　18 gtt/1 mL = ?/15 mL　　　? = 270 drops per bottle
25c　75 mg/270 gtt = ?/1 drop
　　　? = 0.278 mg = 278 mcg/gtt

26a　50 mg nitro/1000 mL = ?/100 mL
　　　? = 5 mg/100 mL = 0.005 g/100 mL = 0.005%
26b　50,000 mcg nitro/1000 mL = 200 mcg nitro/?
　　　? = 4 mL solution

27　5 g drug/100 mL = 0.015 g (test dose)/?
　　　? = 0.3 mL of the 5% sol.

28　200 mg/dL → 200 mg/100 mL → 0.2 g/100 mL → 0.2%

29　0.15% → 0.15 g/100 mL → 150 mg/100 mL →150 mg%
　　or (150 mg/dL)

30　95 mg% → 95 mg/100 mL
　　95 mg cholesterol/100 mL = ?/1 mL
　　　? = 0.95 mg = 950 mcg

31a　8 ppm → 8/1,000,000 → 1/125,000 → 1:125,000
31b　8/1,000,000 = 0.000008 = 0.0008%
31c　8 g antifungal/1,000,000 g feed = ?/1000 g feed
　　　? = 0.008 g antifungal

32　1 g sod. fluoride/1,000,000 mL = ?/3,840,000 mL
　　　? = 3.84 g sodium fluoride

33　0.00005 g/100 mL = ?/1,000,000 mL
　　　? = 0.5 g/1,000,000 = 0.5 ppm

34　0.00005 g/100 mL = ?/1000 mL　　　? = 0.0005 g = 500 mcg

35a　2/7 = 1/?　　　　? = 3.5　　　2:7 → 1:3.5
35b　17/510 = 1/?　　　? = 30　　　17:510 → 1:30
35c　33/135 = 1/?　　　? = 4.1　　　33:135 → 1:4.1
35d　0.125 → 125/1000 → 125:1000 → 1:8
　　　(I just reduced this one, but you can work it either way.)
35e　0.08 → 8/100 → 8:100 → 8/100 = 1/?
　　　? = 12.5　　　　　　　　8:100 → 1:12.5
35f　0.45 → 45/100 = 1/?
　　　? = 2.22　　　　　　　　45:100 → 1:2.22
35g　2:23 → 2/23 = 1/?
　　　? = 11.5　　　　　　　　2:23 → 1:11.5
35h　23:300 → 23/300 = 1/?
　　　? = 13.04　　　　　　　23:300 → 1:13.04
35i　48:200 → 48/200 = 1/?
　　　? = 4.167　　　　　　　48:200 → 1:4.167

NOTE: To check your answers, divide the ratios and see if the
*decimal fractions* are similar. *Example*: for 35i, you would get
48/200 = 0.24 and 1/4.167 = 0.24

36a　6 mg pest/1,000,000 mg = 1 mg pest/?
　　　? = 166,667 mg = 167 g = 0.167 kg
36b　6/1,000,000 = 1/?
　　　? = 166,667 so the ratio is 1:166,667

37a　1 g/1000 mL = ?/3000 mL　　　　? = 3 g
　　　0.5 g/1 tablet = 3 g/?　　　　? = 6 tablets
37b　0.5 g/1 tablet = ?/60 tablets　　? = 30 g
　　　30 g/3000 mL = ?/100 mL
　　　? = 1 g, so this solution provides 1 g/100 mL or 1%

38a　10% × 500 mL = 50 mL of resorcinol monoacetate needed.
38b　10% is the same as a 1:10 ratio strength. Did you remember
　　　that this ratio strength does not change based on the volume?
　　　One liter is 1:10 strength, one drop is 1:10 strength, and
　　　8.35 mL is also a 1:10 ratio strength, or 10%.

39a　0.05 mg/1 mL = ?/100 mL　　　　? = 5 mg
　　　5 mg/100 mL represents a 5 mg% solution
39b　5 mg/100 mL = ?/5 mL　　　　　? = 0.25 mg = 250 mcg

40a　0.5 g/100 mL = ?/30 mL　　　　? = 0.15 g = 150 mg
40b　1 g/200,000 = ?/1 mL
　　　? = 0.000005 g = 0.005 mg = 5 mcg

41a　160 mg = 0.16 g sodium
　　　0.16 sodium:3.2 total weight
　　　0.16/3.2 = 1/?　　　　　　　? = 20
　　　1:20 is the ratio strength of sodium to total weight
41b　250 mg = 0.25 g
　　　0.25 g/3.2 g = 0.078 = 7.8%

42a　0.0025 × 5 mL = 0.0125 g = 12.5 mg
42b　0.25% = 0.25 g:100 mL = 1:400

NOTE: The ratio strength is the same no matter the volume.

43a　5 mg/1 mL = ?/100 mL　　　　　? = 500 mg or 0.5 g
　　　0.5 g/100 mL = 0.5%
43b　5 mg/1 mL = ?/20,000 mL　　　　? = 100,000 mg = 100 g

44a　4% = 4:100 = 1:25

NOTE: The 50- and 100-mL bottles are both 4%, so they are both 1:25.

44b　3 mL × 4% = 0.12 g = 120 mg

45a　0.5 + 0.75 + 1 + 1.5 + 2 + 4 + 6 = 15.75 mg
　　　15.75 mg/30 mL = ?/100 mL　　　? = 52.5
　　　52.5 mg/100 mL = 52.5 mg%
45b　52.5 mg = 0.0525 g
　　　0.0525 g/100 mL = 1/?　　　? = 1905　　　1:1905

# CHAPTER 9

1    12 techs × 100 Rx = 1200 techsRx
     20 techs × 125 Rx = 2500 techsRx
     23 techs × 150 Rx = 3450 techsRx
     __8 techs__ × 175 Rx = __1400 techsRx__
     63 techs                8550 techsRx

     8550 techsRx/63 techs = 135.7 Rx (per tech)
     ("techs" cancel out)

2       2 liters × 20% =   40 liter%
        1 liter  × 50% =   50 liter%
     __0.75 liter__ × 80% = __60 liter%__
     3.75 liters           150 liter%

     (Make sure all units are the same. I selected liters, but mLs are OK.)
     150 liter%/3.75 liters = 40%

NOTE: I frequently see mistakes with this type of problem when students accidentally add the middle column or divide by the wrong numbers. Please be careful.

*(Of course, you would not make a mistake like that, because you always ESTIMATE the correct answer. Right?)*

3      1 pint  × 10% =   10 pint%
       6 pints ×  5% =   30 pint%
     __8 pints__ × 20% = __160 pint%__
     15 pints          200 pint%

     200 pint%/15 pints = 13.33%

4    15 pints × 13.33% = 200 pint%
     __2 pints__ ×     0% = __0 pint%__
     17 pints            200 pint%

     200 pint%/17 pints = 11.76%

5     480 mL × 2% =   960 mL%
     __1000 mL__ × 6% = __6000 mL%__
     1480 mL          6960 mL%

     6960 mL%/1480 mL = 4.7%

6    1480 mL × 4.7% = 6956 mL%
     __500 mL__ × 0.2% = __100 mL%__
     1980 mL           7056 mL%

     7056 mL%/1980 mL = 3.56%

7    1000 mL × 95% = 95,000 mL%
      960 mL × 70% = 67,200 mL%
     __480 mL__ ×  0% = __0 mL%__
     2440 mL          162,200 mL%

     (480 mL is 17% benzalkonium chloride BUT 0% alcohol)
     162,200 mL%/2440 mL = 66.48%

8    5% + 15% + 20% = 40%        40%/3 = 13.33%
     (This is like your English test average, but a lot lower. You can also work this by alligation medial if you wish.)

9    300 grams × 13.33% =   4000 gram%
     __100 grams__ ×    100% = __10,000 gram%__
     400 grams               14,000 gram%

     14,000 gram%/400 grams = 35%

10    454 grams × 2% =   908 gram%
     __1000 grams__ × 5% = __5000 gram%__
     1454 grams           5908 gram%

     5908 gram%/1454 grams = 4.06%

11a  (OV)(O%) = (NV)(N%)
     (30 mL)(10%) = (1000 mL)(N%)        0.3% = N%
11b  0.3% = 0.3/100    0.3/100 = 1/?     ? = 333 → 1:333
11c  0.3 g/100 mL = ?/15 mL
     ? = 0.045 g/tablespoonful
11d  10 g/100 mL = ?/5 mL
     ? = 0.5 g/teaspoonful

12a  (OV)(O%) = (NV)(N%)
     (120)(10%) = (NV)(1%)        1200 mL = NV
12b  1200 mL − 120 mL = 1080 mL
     of diluent to be added to the 120 mL of 10% stock

13   (OV)(O%) = (NV)(N%)
     (OV)(17%) = (1000)(0.5%)        OV = 29.4 mL

14   0.5 g/100 mL = ?/30 mL        ? = 0.15 gram = 150 mg

15   (OV)(O%) = (NV)(N%)
     (10)(O%) = (1000)(0.5%)        O% = 50%

16   50 g/100 mL = ?/480 mL
     ? = 240 grams in the 50% stock bottle

17a  (OV)(O%) = (NV)(N%)
     (1 oz)(5%) = (5 oz)(N%)        1% = N%

NOTE: We added 4 oz to the 1 oz of 5% = 5 oz total.

17b  1% = 1/100 = 1:100

18   (OV)(O%) = (NV)(N%)
     (OV)(2%) = (960)(0.05%)        OV = 24 mL

19   (OV)(O%) = (NV)(N%)
     (480)(95%) = (NV)(20%)        2280 mL = NV

NOTE: This is the *final* dilution, but it is not the answer to the question. If we started with a pint and finished with 2280 mL, then we had to add a diluent to the pint to get 2280 mL. The correct volume that was *added* is 2280 − 480 = 1800 mL.

20a  (OV) (O%) = (NV) (N%)
(100) (50%) = (500) (N%)          10% = N%

NOTE: Again, 400 mL was *added* to 100 mL to make a final volume of 500 mL. Be very careful in reading these dilution questions.

20b  (OV) (O%) = (NV) (N%)
(100) (50%) = (NV) (5%)          1000 mL = NV
20c  1000 mL − 100 mL = 900 mL to be added
20d  (OV) (O%) = (NV) (N%)
(100) (50%) = (1100) (N%)

NOTE: You are adding 100 mL of 50% + dextrose to 1000 mL of 0% dextrose. The latter solution is 0.9% NaCl, but 0% dextrose. 4.55% = N%

21  *GOTCHA!* You cannot add a 6% ointment and a 50% ointment to make a 4% ointment. As mentioned earlier, your answer has to be between the 6% and 50% ointments in concentration.

22a  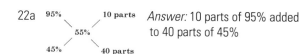  *Answer:* 10 parts of 95% added to 40 parts of 45%

22b  Total parts equal 50 parts of the 55% final product
(i.e., 10 + 40 = 50)          50 parts/1000 mL = 10 parts/?
? = 200 mL of the 95% alcohol
22c  50 parts/1000 mL = 40 parts/?
? = 800 mL of the 45% alcohol

NOTE: The shortcut is: 1000 mL final product − 200 mL of the 95% solution = 800 mL.

22d  This question is limited by the quantity in least supply, in this case, 1 pint of 95% alcohol.
10 parts/480 mL = 50 parts/?
? = 2400 mL of 55% alcohol can be made

23a  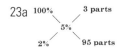  *Answer:* 3 parts of 100% added to 95 parts of 2%

23b  98 parts/454 g = 95 parts/?
? = 440.1 g of the 2% coal tar needed
23c  454 − 440.1 = 13.9 g of the 100% coal tar needed
(Can also be done with ratios.)
23d  3 parts/113.5 g = 98 parts/?
? = 3707.7 g = 3.708 kg

24a  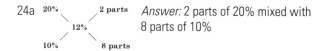  *Answer:* 2 parts of 20% mixed with 8 parts of 10%

24b  10 parts/480 mL = 8 parts/?
? = 384 mL of the 10% solution
24c  12 g/100 mL = ?/480 mL
? = 57.6 g KCl/pint of 12%

24d  12 g/100 mL = ?/15 mL
? = 1.8 g = 1800 mg
24e  You can work this by alligation, but, since you are using a zero percent diluent, you can also work this as a simple dilution:
(OV) (O%) = (NV) (N%)
(OV) (20%) = (1000) (12%)          OV = 600 mL of the 20%
*Answer:* 1000 − 600 = 400 mL diluent

25a  YES, you can mix a 20% solution with a 1% solution and make an intermediate strength of 2%.
25b  1 part × 20% = 20 part%
1 part × 1% = 1 part%
2 parts          21 part%

21 part%/2 parts = 10.5% lidocaine

25c  30 mL × 1% = 30 mL%
20 mL × 20% = 400 mL%
50 mL          430 mL%

430 mL%/50 mL = 8.6% lidocaine

25d  0.4 g/100 mL = ?/1 mL
? = 0.004 g = 4 mg
25e  30 mL/1 hr = ?/24 hr
? = 720 mL of 5% dextrose in 24 hours
5 g/100 mL = ?/720 mL
? = 36 g of dextrose per day

26a  1 g antifungal/750 g cream = ?/1 g cream
? = 0.00133 g = 1.33 mg
26b  1:750 is equal to 0.133%
Solved by the old-volume old-percent method:
NV = 178 g (60 + 118)
(118 g) (0.133%) = (178 g) (?)          ? = 0.088%

Solved by the alligation medial method
118 g × 0.133% = 15.694 g%
60 g × 0% = 0 g%
178 g          15.694 g%

15.694 g%/178 g = 0.088%

27a  25 gtt/1 mL = 20 gtt/?
? = 0.8 mL 10 g/100 mL = ?/0.8 mL    ? = 0.08 g = 80 mg
27b  Solved by old-volume old-percent, with the final volume
5.8 mL (5 + 0.8)
(0.8 mL) (10%) = (5.8 mL) (?)          ? = 1.38%

28a  1 mL cinn. oil/400 mL = 35 mL cinn. oil/?
? = 14,000 mL = 14 L
28b  Solved by old-volume old-percent method:
1:400 is the same as 0.25%, and the new volume is 135 mL (35 + 100). Consider the oil to be 100%. (35 mL) (100%)
= (135 mL) (?)          ? = 25.9%
Can also be solved by alligation medial using alcohol as 0% cinnamon oil.

29a  500 mg = 0.5 g     10 g/100 mL = 0.5 g/?    ? = 5 mL
29b  0.5 g/30 mL = 1 g/?        ? = 60 mL
     1 g in 60 mL is a 1:60 ratio strength

30a  2.5 g/10 mL = ?/100 mL     ? = 25 g
     (25 g/100 mL = 25%)
30b  10 mL × 25% = 250%
     $\underline{50\ mL\ \times\ \ \ 5\% = \ \ 250\ mL\%}$
     60 mL                 500 mL%

     500 mL%/60 mL = 8.33%

31a  1 mg/0.2 mL = ?/100 mL    ? = 500 mg = 0.5 g
     0.5 g/100 mL = 0.5%
31b  (OV) (O%) = (NV) (N%)
     (0.4 mL) (0.5%) = (60 mL) (?)    ? = 0.0033%

32a  500 mg/2.2 mL = ?/1 mL    ? = 227 mg/mL
32b  5 mL + 2.2 mL = 7.2 mL
     500 mg/7.2 mL = ?/1 mL    ? = 69.4 mg/mL

33a  5 mcg/1 mL = ?/100 mL    ? = 500 mcg = 0.5 mg =
     0.0005 g per 100 mL = 0.0005%
33b  300 mcg/mL = ?/100 mL    ? = 30,000 mcg = 30 mg
     = 0.03 g per 100 mL = 0.03%
     (OV) (O%) = (NV) (N%)
     (1 mL) (0.03%) = (?) (0.0005%)    ? = 60 mL
     60 mL − 1 mL means you can add 59 mL

34a  1.5-g vial contains 0.5 g sulbactam
     3-g vial contains 1 g sulbactam
     0.5 g + 1 g + 1 g + 1 g = 3.5 g sulbactam
34b  2 g ampicillin/8 mL = 0.25 = 25%

35a  Adding 2% creams to 2% creams yields a final cream that is 2%.
35b  You cannot add 100% ketoconazole to a 2% cream and get a
     lower percent strength. The percent strength will only increase.

# CHAPTER 10

1a  10 g KCl/100 mL = ?/480 mL    ? = 48 grams KCl/pint
1b  MW KCl = 74.5
     valence = 1, so 74.5 mg/1 = 74.5 mg per mEq
     74.5 mg/1 mEq = 48,000 mg/?    ? = 644.3 mEq KCl/pint
1c  644.3 mEq potassium (see "statement of unity" discussion)
1d  644.3 mEq KCl/480 mL = ?/15 mL
     ? = 20.1 mEq KCl/tablespoon
1e  10 mEq q.i.d. = 40 mEq daily
     644.3 mEq/480 mL = 40 mEq/?    ? = 29.8 mL = 30 mL

2a  MW NaCl = 58.5, and valence = 1,
     so 58.5 mg/1 = 58.5 mg per mEq
     58.5 mg/1 mEq = 1000 mg/?
     ? = 17.1 mEq NaCl per tablet
2b  1 tab × 3 × 7 days = 21 tablets
     1 tablet/17.1 mEq = 21 tablets/?
     ? = 359 mEq NaCl → 359 mEq Na

2c  17.1 mEq Na/1 tab = 100 mEq Na/?
     ? = 5.84 tablets = 6 tablets

3  1 mEq NaCl/58.5 mg = 154 mEq NaCl/?
   ? = 9009 mg = 9.009 grams NaCl

4  9.009 g/1000 mL = ?/100 mL
   ? = 0.9 g/100 mL = 0.9% (normal saline)

5a  1 mEq NaCl = 58.5 mg    1 mEq Na/1 kg = ?/72 kg
     ? = 72 mEq
     1 mEq NaCl/58.5 mg = 72 mEq NaCl/?
     ? = 4212 mg NaCl
5b  1 mEq/2.2 lb = ?/110 lb    ? = 50 mEq NaCl
     1 mEq NaCl/58.5 mg = 50 mEq/?
     ? = 2925 mg = 2.925 g
5c  0.9 g NaCl/100 mL = 2.925 g NaCl/?   ? = 325 mL of NS
5d  14.6 g NaCl/100 mL = 2.925 g NaCl/?
     ? = 20 mL of 14.6% NaCl

6  100 mL/1 hr = ?/24 hr    ? = 2400 mL daily
   0.9 g NaCl/100 mL = ?/2400 mL   ? = 21.6 g NaCl daily
   58.5 mg NaCl/1 mEq = 21,600 mg NaCl/?
   ? = 369 mEq Na daily

7a  MW $CaCl_2$ = 111        valence = 2,
     so 111 mg/2 = 55.5 mg per mEq
     1 mEq $CaCl_2$/55.5 mg = 30 mEq $CaCl_2$/?   ? = 1665 mg $CaCl_2$
7b  1.665 g/1000 mL = ?/100 mL
     ? = 0.1665% calcium chloride

8a  MW $NaHCO_3$ = 84      valence = 1,
     so 84 mg/1 = 84 mg per mEq
     90 mEq/100 mL = ?/1000 mL   ? = 900 mEq
     1 mEq/84 mg = 900 mEq/?   ? = 75,600 mg/L
8b  75.6 g/1000 mL = ?/100 mL   ? = 7.56%

9a  MW $NH_4Cl$ = 53.5      valence = 1,
     so 53.5 mg/1 = 53.5 mg per mEq
     1 mEq/53.5 mg = 100 mEq/?
     ? = 5350 mg = 5.35 g
     5.35 g/20 mL = ?/100 mL
     ? = 26.75% ammonium chloride
9b  5.35 g/520 mL = ?/100 mL   ? = 1.03%
     (500 + 20 = 520 mL)

10a  MW $NaC_2H_3O_2$ = 82    valence = 1,
     so 82 mg/1 = 82 mg per mEq
     1 mEq/82 mg = 4 mEq/?   ? = 328 mg per mL
     328 mg/1 mL = 1000 mg/?   ? = 3.05 mL
10b  4 mEq/1 mL = ?/5 mL    ? = 20 mEq of sodium
     acetate = 20 mEq sodium (see "statement of unity")
10c  0.328 g/1 mL = ?/100 mL   ? = 32.8%

11a  4.2 g/100 mL = ?/10 mL   ? = 0.42 g = 420 mg
11b  0.5 mEq/1 mL = ?/10 mL
     ? = 5 mEq sodium bicarbonate

11c The 420 mg in item (a) gives the total weight of sodium bicarbonate in the syringe. Your answer in item (b) indicates how many mEq of sodium bicarbonate are in the syringe, so you have all the information needed.
420 mg/5 mEq = ?/1 mEq          ? = 84 mg
11d 1 mEq/84 mg = 2.5 mEq/?          ? = 210 mg = 0.21 g
0.21 g/1 mL = ?/100 mL
? = 21 g (21 g/100 mL = 21%)

12a 0.8 mEq/1 mL = ?/480 mL          ? = 384 mEq
1 mEq/74.5 mg = 384 mEq/?          ? = 28,608 mg = 28.61 g
12b Using the answer in item (a)
28.61 g/480 mL = ?/100 mL
? = 5.96 g per 100 mL or 5.96%

13a Daily dose is 5 mL q.i.d. or 20 mL
5 g/100 mL = ?/20 mL          ? = 1 g = 1000 mg daily
1 mEq = 111/2 = 55.5 mg
1 mEq/55.5 mg = ?/1000 mg          ? = 18 mEq/day
13b 5 g/100 mL = ?/240 mL          ? = 12 g = 12,000 mg
1 mEq/55.5 mg = ?/12,000 mg          ? = 216.2 mEq

14a 2 mEq/1 mL = ?/20 mL          ? = 40 mEq
1 mEq/74.5 = 40 mEq/?          ? = 2980 mg = 2.98 g
2.98 g/20 mL = ?/100 mL
? = 14.9 g per 100 mL = 14.9%
14b. Use the answer from item (a)
(OV) (O%) = (NV) (N%)
(20 mL)(14.9%) = (1000 mL)(?)          ? = 0.298%

15a 50 mg/1 mL = ?/6 mL          ? = 300 mg = 0.3 g
15b 300 mg/1 day = ?/3 days          ? = 900 mg
1 mEq = 274/1 = 274 mg          1 mEq/274 mg = ?/900 mg
? = 3.28 mEq phenytoin sodium and 3.28 mEq sodium

16a 50 mEq/50 mL = ?/1 mL          ? = 1 mEq per mL
1 mEq = 84/1 = 84 mg          84 mg/mL
16b 84 mg/1 mL = ?/100 mL
? = 8400 mg = 8.4 g per 100 mL = 8.4%
16c There are 50 mEq of sodium bicarbonate in a syringe. If 1 mEq of sodium bicarbonate yields 1 mEq of sodium, then there are 50 mEq of sodium in the syringe.
16d There are 50 mEq of sodium bicarbonate per 50 mL of the solution, so there is 1 mEq in 1 mL. 1 mEq sodium bicarbonate yields 1 mEq sodium and 1 mEq bicarbonate, so the answer is 1 mEq.

17a 10 g/100 mL = 2 g/?
? = 20 mL of the 10% injection
17b 10 mL calcium gluconate + 100 mL sodium chloride = 110 mL (final volume)
(OV) (O%) = (NV) (N%)
(10 mL) (10%) = (110 mL) (?)          ? = 0.91%
17c 50 mL × 10% = 5 g calcium gluconate = 5000 mg
1 mEq calcium gluconate = 430/2 = 215 mg

NOTE: 1 mEq calcium gluconate yields 1 mEq calcium.
1 mEq/215 mg = ?/5000 mg
? = 23.26 mEq of calcium gluconate and calcium/50 mL

17d From the answer to item (c), there are 23.26 mEq calcium per 50 mL.
23.26 mEq/50 mL = ?/2 mL          ? = 0.93 mEq/2 mL dose

# CHAPTER 11

1a °C = (°F − 32) ÷ 1.8 (Use this formula for 1a–1e.)
= (41 − 32) ÷ 1.8 = 9 ÷ 1.8 = 5°C
1b = (86 − 32) ÷ 1.8 = 54 ÷ 1.8 = 30°C
1c = (167 − 32) ÷ 1.8 = 135 ÷ 1.8 = 75°C
1d = (14 − 32) ÷ 1.8 = (−18) ÷ 1.8 = − 10°C
1e = (− 40 − 32) ÷ 1.8 = (−72) ÷ 1.8 = − 40°C (same value)

2a °F = (1.8 × °C) + 32 (Use this formula for 2a–2e.)
= (1.8 × 15) + 32 = (27) + 32 = 59°F
2b = (1.8 × 75) + 32 = 135 + 32 = 167°F
2c = (1.8 × 0) + 32 = 0 + 32 = 32°F
2d = (1.8 × −5) + 32 = − 9 + 32 = 23°F
2e = (1.8 × −75) + 32 = −135 + 32 = − 103°F

3 (1.8 × −20) + 32 = (− 36) + 32 = −4°F

4 (23 − 32) ÷ 1.8 = (− 9) ÷ 1.8 = −5°C

5 (1.8 × 60) + 32 = (108) + 32 = 140°F

6 (177 − 32) ÷ 1.8 = (145) ÷ 1.8 = 80.6°C

7 (1.8 × −15) + 32 = (−27) + 32 = 5°F

8 (−58 − 32) ÷ 1.8 = (−90) ÷ 1.8 = −50°C

9 (1.8 × 30) + 32 = (54) + 32 = 86°F

10 (40 − 32) ÷ 1.8 = (8) ÷ 1.8 = 4.4°C

11 (1.8 × −111) + 32 = (−199.8) + 32 = −168°F

12 (98.6 − 32) ÷ 1.8 = (66.6) ÷ 1.8 = 37°C

13a °F = (1.8 × 2) + 32 = 35.6°F
°F = (1.8 × 8) + 32 = 46.4°F
Range is 36°F to 46°F.
13b Store in the refrigerator.

14a °C = (68 − 32) ÷ 1.8 = 20°C
°C = (77 − 32) ÷ 1.8 = 25°C
Range is 20°C to 25°C.
14b Store at USP controlled room temperature.

15 °F = (1.8 × 25) + 32 = 77°F
The label states to not freeze, so it must be stored at a temperature above 32°F but no warmer than 77°F.

# CHAPTER 12

1a   $78 − $45 = $33 markup
1b   ($78 − $45)/$78 = 33/78 = 0.42 = 42%
      markup based on selling price
1c   ($78 − $45)/$45 = 33/45 = 0.73 = 73%
      markup based on cost
1d   1.72 × $45 = $77.40
      (selling price based on 72% markup on cost)
1e   100% − 72% = 28% (cost of the product)
      28%/100% = $45/?                        ? = $160.71
      (selling price based on 72% markup on selling price)

2a   $78 − $12 = $66
2b   $78/60 tablets = ?/1 tablet        ? = $1.30 per tablet
2c   $12/60 tablets = ?/1 tablet        ? = $0.20
2d   1 tablet × 2 × 7 days = 14 tablets/wk
      60 tablets/$78 = 14 tablets/?        ? = $18.20
2e   (78 − 66)/66 = 12/66 = 0.182 = 18.2% markup based on *cost*
2f   (78 − 66)/78 = 12/78 = 0.154 = 15.4% markup based on
      *selling price*

3a   GP = sales − cost = $4,300,000 − $2,670,000 = $1,630,000
3b   NP = GP − overhead = $1,630,000 − $850,000 = $780,000
3c   100%/$780,000 = 5%/?                    ? = $39,000
      (If you don't want it, I'll take it!)
3d   Inventory turnover rate = total purchases/average inventory
      ITR = $2,670,000/$520,000 = 5.13 times
3e   $62/1 sale = $4,300,000/?        ? = 69,355 total sales

4a   $81,435 − $69,887 = $11,548 monthly gross profit
4b   Think about this. If the *gross* profit is $11,548 and the *net* profit is
      $5,328, then the *overhead* is the difference in these two numbers.
      Remember that net profit is gross profit minus overhead.
      $11,548 − $5328 = $6220 overhead

5a   1.20 × $331 = $397.20
      (the amount 100 tablets would cost with markup)
      100 tablets/$397.20 = 30 tablets/?        ? = $119.16

NOTE: You could also take the *cost* of 30 tablets ($99.30) and
multiply by 1.2 and get the same answer.

5b   100% total cost *after* markup − 10% markup =
      90% *original cost* of the drug
      90% (cost) /$331 = 100% (selling price)/?        ? = $367.78

NOTE: To check your answer, subtract 10% of the *selling price* from
the selling price, and your answer (hopefully) will be the original
cost. ($367.78 − $36.78 = $331)

5b   $367.78/100 tablets  = ?/60 tablets
      ? = $220.67

5c   $331 × 0.92 = $304.52 or
      100%/$331 = 92%/?                    ? = $304.52

6a   $14.88/12 tubes = ?/1 tube        ? = $1.24 (cost for
      1 tube) markup = $2.69 − $1.24 = $1.45
6b   ($2.69 − $1.24)/$2.69 = $1.45/$2.69 = 0.54 = 54%
6c   ($2.69 − $1.24)/$1.24 = $1.45/$1.24 = 1.17 = 117%
6d   100% − 30% = 70% (amount a customer will pay after the
      30% discount) 100%/$2.69 = 70%/?   ? = $1.88
      Alternate solution: 70%/100% = ?/$2.69    ? = $1.88
      Or just multiply: 70% × $2.69 = 0.7 × $2.69 = $1.88
6e   1 tube/$1.24 = 3 tubes/?              ? = $3.72 (cost of 3 tubes)
      Markup = 185% × $3.72 = $6.88 (markup on the 3 tubes)
      Alternate solution: 100%/$3.72 = 185%/?    ? = $6.88
      Final price = cost + markup = $3.72 + $6.88 = $10.60

7a   Selling price = 100% (cost) + 40% (markup) = 140%
      140%/$38.35 = 100%/?                    ? = $27.39 (original cost)
      Check answer: % markup = (selling price − cost)/cost
      = % markup = ($38.35 − $27.39)/$27.39 = 0.4 = 40%
7b   Markup = selling price − cost = $38.35 − $27.39 (from 7a)
      = $10.96        $10.96/30 tablets = ?/1 tablet
      ? = $0.37 markup per tablet

8    100% − 40% = 60% (the final cost after the 40% discount)
      100%/$27.85 = 60%/?
      ? = $16.71 (cost per gallon after discount)
      Alternate solution:
      60% × $27.85 = 0.6 × $27.85 = $16.71
      $16.71/8 pints = ?/1 pint
      ? = $2.09 (cost per pint after discount)

9    12 × 10 doses = 120 doses
      $1068/120 doses = ?/1 dose
      ? = $8.90 (cost for each vaccine)
      Final price = cost + markup = $8.90 + $16 = $24.90

10   1 kg/2.2 lb = ?/110 lb
      ? = 50 kg (patient's weight)
      0.2 mg/1 kg = ?/50 kg              ? = 10 mg (daily dose)
      $46.50/20 mg = ?/10 mg              ? = $23.25 (cost per day)

11a  3 tablets/day = ?/10 days            ? = 30 tablets
      100 tablets/$115.85 = 30 tablets/?    ? = $34.76
11b  $115.85 is 93% of the original price before the discount,
      so the original price is 100%.
      $115.85/93% = ?/100%              ? = $124.57
      $124.57/100 tablets = ?/60 tablets    ? = $74.74

12a  60 tablets × 5 bottles = 300 tablets
      $305/300 tablets = ?/1 tablet        ? = $1.02
12b  2 × 2 × 7 = 28 tablets to be dispensed
      1 tablet/$1.02 = 28 tablets/?        ? = $28.56
12c  cost + 4% + $3 = ?
      cost = $28.56 from item (b)
      4% = 0.04 × $28.56 = $1.14
      $28.56 + $1.14 + $3 = $32.70
      $32.70 − cost = profit            $32.70 − $28.56 = $4.14

# CHAPTER 13

1    375 mg/5 mL = 500 mg/?        ? = 6.7 mL

2    0.5 mg = 500 mcg
     500 mcg/1 tablet = 62.5 mcg/?
     ? = 0.125 or 1/8 tablet

3    80 mg/2 mL = 100 mg/?         ? = 2.5 mL

4    60 mEq/4 doses = ?/1 dose     ? = 15 mEq per dose
     20 mEq/15 mL = 15 mEq/?       ? = 11.25 mL

5    2000 mg/4 doses = ?/1 dose    ? = 500 mg per dose
     62.5 mg/5 mL = 500 mg/?       ? = 40 mL

6    50 mcg/1 mL = 75 mcg/?        ? = 1.5 mL

7    7 hours = 420 min
     1000 mL/420 min = ?/1 min     ? = 2.38 mL/min
     10 gtt/1 mL = ?/2.38 mL       ? = 23.8 = 24 gtt/min

8    Vistaril 25 mg , 25 mg/1 mL, so 1 mL is needed
     Demerol 25 mg, 50 mg/1 mL, so 1/2 mL needed
     1 mL Vistaril + 1/2 mL Demerol = 1 1/2 mL total volume

9    100 mL/30 min = ?/60 min      ? = 200 mL/hr

10   15 gtt/1 mL = 50 gtt/?        ? = 3.33 mL/min
     3.33 mL/1 min = 90 mL/?       ? = 27 min
     Alternate method:
     15 gtt/1 mL = ?/90 mL         ? = 1350 gtt total
     50 gtt/1 min = 1350 gtt/?     ? = 27 min

11   30 mL/60 min = 250 mL/?
     ? = 500 min or 8 hr + 20 min
     1900 hours is the same as 7 p.m.
     Add 8 hours and 20 minutes to get
     0320 hours, which is the same as 3:20 a.m.

12   25,000 units/500 mL = ?/20 mL      ? = 1000 units per hour

13   2000 mg/250 mL = 2 mg/?
     ? = 0.25 mL/min or 15 mL/hr

14   8 mL/60 min = ?/1 min         ? = 0.1333 mL/min
     50 mg/250 mL = ?/0.1333 mL
     ? = 0.0267 mg = 26.7 mcg/min

15   100 mL/120 min = ?/1 min      ? = 0.833 mL/min

16   50 mL × 6 = 300 mL daily provided by the formula
     30 mL × 4 = 120 mL daily provided by the medication
     300 + 120 = 420 mL daily provided daily by the formula
     and the medication

17   500,000 units/1 mL = 2,500,000 units/?      ? = 5 mL

18   1 mg/1 min = 60 mg/?          ? = 60 min
     2 mg/1 min = 60 mg/?          ? = 30 min
     The range is 30 to 60 minutes.

19   1 kg/2.2 lb = ?/55            ? = 25 kg (child's weight)
     50 mg/1 kg = ?/25 kg          ? = 1250 mg

20   20 units/500 mL = 3 units/?   ? = 75 mL/hr

21   40 g/1000 mL = 3.5 g/?        ? = 87.5 mL/hr

22a  final volume – diluent = dry powder volume
     35 mL – 24 mL = 11 mL
22b  10 mg/1 mL = ?/35 mL          ? = 350 mg = 0.35 g
22c  1 kg/2.2 lb = ?/48 lb         ? = 21.8 kg (child's weight)
     3 mg/ 1 kg = ?/21.8 kg        ? = 65.4 mg dose needed
     10 mg/1 mL = 65.4 mg/?        ? = 6.54 or 6.5 mL needed

23a  400 mg/250 mL = ?/15 mL       ? = 24 mg = 0.024 g
23b  1 kg/2.2 lb = ?/163 lb
     ? = 74.1 kg (patient's weight)
     24,000 mcg/60 min = ?/1 min   ? = 400 mcg/min
     400 mcg/74.1 kg = ?/1 kg      ? = 5.4 mcg/kg/min
23c  15 mL/60 min = 250 mL/?       ? = 1000 min

24   0.02 g/100 mL = ?/2.5 mL      ? = 0.0005 g = 0.5 mg

25a  1 kg/2.2 lb = ?/8.2 lb
     ? = 3.73 kg (baby's weight)
     0.05 mg/1 kg = ?/3.73 kg      ? = 0.187 mg dose
     6 mg/2 mL = 0.187 mg/?        ? = 0.062 mL dose
25b  0.003 g = 3 mg                3 mg/10 mL = 0.187 mg/?
     ? = 0.62 mL dose

## PI Challenge

26   60 minutes/1 hr = ?/24 hr     ? = 1440 min/day
     0.5 mg/1 min = ?/1440 min     ? = 720 mg = 0.72 g/day

27   1936 × 14% = 271 patients received the investigational drug
     or 14 patients/100 patients = ?/1936 patients
     ? = 271 patients

28   10 g/100 mL = 0.2 g/?         ? = 2 mL

29   100 mg/capsule = 600 mg/?     ? = 6 capsules/day
     6 capsules/1 day = ?/7 days   ? = 42 capsules/week

30   4 × 1.7 = 6.8 mcg/mL
     or 1 mg (inj)/4 mcg (conc) = 1.7 mg (inj)/?
     ? = 6.8 mcg/mL concentration

31   176 lb/2.2 = 80 kg            1 mg/kg = ?/80 kg
     ? = 80 mg q.8h = 240 mg/day   80 mg/1 vial = 240 mg/?
     ? = 3 vials

32  0.02% = 0.02 g/100 mL
    0.02 g/100 mL = ?/2.5 mL          ? = 0.0005 g = 0.5 mg/vial

33  198 lb/2.2 = 90 kg               2 mg/1 kg = ?/90 kg
    ? = 180-mg dose of methylene blue

34  1 mg/3 days = ?/1 day
    ? = 0.333 mg = 333 mcg/day

35  154 lb/2.2 = 70 kg               0.6 mg/1 kg = ?/70 kg
    ? = 42 mg                         20 mg/1 mL = 42 mg/?
    ? = 2.1 mL of succinylcholine chloride injection

36  Degrees Fahrenheit = (1.8 × 2) + 32 = 35.6°F
    Degrees Fahrenheit = (1.8 × 8) + 32 = 46.4°F
    36 to 46°F would require refrigeration
    (below 32°F would need to be frozen)

37  1 mL/1 min = ?/25 min            ? = 25 mL
    1 g/50 mL = ?/25 mL
    ? = 0.5 g = 500 mg of procainamide hydrochloride

38  10 mcg/1 mL = ?/1000 mL
    ? = 10,000 mcg = 10 mg = 0.01 g/liter

39  6.6 lb/2.2 = 3 kg                10 mcg/1 kg = ?/3 kg
    ? = 30 mcg = 0.03 mg of levothyroxine sodium

40  1 g/1000 mL = ?/0.5 mL
    ? = 0.0005 g = 0.5 mg of epinephrine

41  Loading dose minimum = 50,000 IU
    800 IU/1 day = ?/14 days
    ? = 11,200 IU over 14 days
    11,200 + 50,000 = ?               ? = 61,200 IU of vitamin D

42a 500 mg/dose × 3 doses/day × 6 days = 9000 mg
    = 9 g of mesalamine
42b 9000 mg × 12% = 1080 mg 5–ASA eliminated in urine over
    6 days

43  If 12 tablets equal the maximum dose, then half of the "max"
    dose is six tablets. 0.125 mg/1 tablet = ?/6 tablets
    ? = 0.75 mg = 750 mcg

44  60 min/1 hr = ?/24 hr            ? = 1440 min/day
    0.75 mg/min = ?/1440 min
    ? = 1080 mg = 1.08 g of clindamycin

45  5 lb/2.2 = 2.27 kg               15 mg/1 kg = ?/2.27 kg
    ? = 34 mg daily/4 doses = 8.5 mg/dose

46  Degrees centigrade = (86 − 32) ÷ 1.8 = 30°C
    Store at room temperature, not in refrigerator.

47  Azithromycin 323/340 = 0.95 = 95%
    Penicillin V 242/332 = 0.73 = 73%
    Azithromycin was 22 percentage points more effective than
    penicillin V.

48  2.5 mg + 25 mg + 2 mg = 29.5 mg/tablet (daily dose)
    29.5 mg/1 day = ?/30 days        ? = 885 mg = 0.885 g

49a Two 20–mL vials = 40 mL added to 260 mL
    = a total volume of 300 mL        5 mg/1 mL = ?/40 mL
    ? = 200 mg labetalol in the two 20–mL vials
    200 mg/300 mL = ?/1 mL
    ? = 0.667 mg of labetalol/mL
49b 2 mg/1 min = ?/30 min            ? = 60 mg/30 min
    0.667 mg/1 mL = 60 mg/?           ? = 90 mL/30 min

50a 200 mcg/1 mL = ?/5 mL            ? = 1000 mcg = 1 mg
50b 5 mg = 0.005 g/mL                0.005 g/1 mL = ?/100 mL
    ? = 0.5 g = 0.5% phenol

51  12%/87 patients = 100%/?          ? = 725 patients
    Check: 87/725 = 0.12 = 12%

52  1 suppository twice daily for 14 days = 28 suppositories
    25 mg/1 suppository = ?/28 suppositories
    ? = 700 mg in 28 suppositories
    700 mg × 26% = 182 mg absorbed

53  50 g/100 mL = ?/1 mL             ? = 0.5 g = 500 mg

54  1 g/5000 mL = 0.0002 g/?         ? = 1 mL

55  5 units/0.25 mL = ?/0.5 mL       ? = 10 units per dose

    NOTE: 5% is equal to 5 units/100 units excreted
    5 units/100 units = ?/10 units
    ? = 0.5 unit excreted in urine
    or 5% excreted × 10 units (dose) = 0.5 unit excreted in urine

56  11/3348 = 0.00328 = 0.33%

57  1% × 336 = 3.36 patients or 3 patients on placebo
    5% × 339 = 16.95 patients or 17 patients on doxazosin
    17 − 3 = 14 more patients receiving doxazosin experienced
    somnolence

58a 200 mg/1 day = ?/7 days = 1400 mg initial daily dose for
    1 week followed by 80 mg × 15 = 1200 mg
    (i.e., 80 mg every other day for 1 month)
    1400 mg + 1200 mg = 2600 mg = 2.6 g of prednisolone
58b 4 mg methylpred/5 mg pred = ?/1400 mg of prednisolone
    ? = 1120 mg = 1.12 g

59  Week 1 = 2 capsules daily for 7 days = 14 capsules
    Week 2 = 4 capsules daily for 7 days = 28 capsules
    14 + 28 = 42 capsules needed for 2 weeks

60   12 gtt/1 mL = ?/5 mL                          ? = 60 gtt/teaspoonful
     4 mg/60 gtt = ?/1 gtt
     ? = 0.0667 mg/drop = 66.7 mcg/drop

61   Since the final concentration is 2 mg/mL, the vial must be
     10 mL in volume to contain 20 total milligrams of the drug.
     If you add 10 mL of diluent to get a final volume of 10 mL,
     there is negligible dry powder volume, and the answer is zero.

62a  The baby weighs 7.19 lb.

NOTE:  3 ounces/16 ounces/lb = 0.19 lb
       7.19 lb/2.2 = 3.27 kg
       15 mg/1 kg = ?/3.27 kg                      ? = 49.1 mg (initial dose)

62b  10 mg/1 kg = ?/3.27 kg
     ? = 32.7 mg q.12h (subsequent doses)
62c  50 mg/1 mL = 49 mg/?
     ? = 0.98 mL = 1 mL (initial dose)
62d  50 mg/1 mL = 32.7 mg/?
     ? = 0.65mL (for subsequent doses)
     0.65 mL/1 dose = ?/2 doses
     ? = 1.3 mL daily (0.65 mL q.12h)

63   Max dose is 3 mL/min = ?/60 min
     ? = 180 mL
     4 g/250 mL = ?/180 mL
     ? = 2.88 g = 2880 mg

64   6.6 lb/2.2 = 3 kg (patient's weight)
     3 mL/1 kg = ?/3 kg                            ? = 9 mL total dose
     35 mg/1 mL = ?/9 mL
     ? = 315 mg of phospholipids

65   1000 g/1 kg = 185 g/?
     ? = 0.185 kg — the weight of a very fat rat!
     150 mg/kg = ?/0.185 kg
     ? = 27.75 mg/day for this specific rat
     27.75 mg/1 day = ?/365 days
     ? = 10,129 mg = 10.13 g of drug per year

66   10,000 × 80 = 800,000 g of product in the large tubes
     0.025 g/100 g = ?/800,000 g
     ? = 200 g of triamcinolone
     Check: 200 g triam./800,000 g total weight = 0.00025 = 0.025%
     454 g/1 lb = 200 g/?
     ? = 0.44 lb of triamcinolone

67   Weeks 1 through 4 = 28 days          1 tab/1 day = ?/28 days
     ? = 28 tablets
     Weeks 5 through 8 = 28 days          2 tabs/1 day = ?/28 days
     ? = 56 tablets
     28 + 56 = 84 tablets for the 8–week titration

68   0.4 mg/day = ?/30 days
     ? = 12 mg of tamsulosin administered
     12 mg × 90% = 10.8 mg absorbed over 30 days

69   50 mcg × 3 = 150 mcg = 0.15 mg (recommended daily dose)
     2.5 mg ÷ 0.15 mg = 16.67 times more than the recommended dose

70a  4.06 mEq/1 mL = ?/10 mL                       ? = 40.6 mEq
     1 mEq = 246/2 = 123 mg
     1 mEq/123 mg = 40.6 mEq/?                      ? = 4994 mg
70b  4994 mg is approximately 5000 mg, or 5 g
     5 g/10 mL = 0.5 = 50%

71   2 mg/500 mL is the same as 2000 mcg/500 mL
     2000 mcg/500 mL = 5 mcg/?                      ? = 1.25 mL

NOTE: When adding quantities like the 10 mL of isoproterenol
to large volumes like the 500 mL of dextrose injection, most
compounders will draw out 10 mL of the 5% dextrose injection
so that the final volume will still be 500 mL. Failure to do this
process will lead to a final volume of 510 mL.
Example: 2000 mcg/510 mL = 5 mcg/?       ? = 1.275 mL

72   1 fold = 100%
     1 fold/100% = 3.2-fold/?                       ? = 320%

73   1 kg/2.2 lb = 23 kg/?
     ? = 50.6 = 51 lb (patient's weight)
     1 mg/1 lb = ?/51 lb                            ? = 51 mg (dose)
     51 mg/2 doses = 25.5 mg/dose

74a  2.5 mg/0.5 mL = ?/100 mL
     ? = 500 mg = 0.5 g/100 mL or 0.5%
     You could also solve it this way:
     0.0025 g/0.5 mL = 0.005 = 0.5%
74b  0.5 g/100 mL = 1/?                             ? = 200 mL
     1/200 = 1:200

75   1/10,000 = ?/3,870,000
     ? = 387 cases of hepatitis

76   Step 1: 1 mEq = 84/1 = 84 mg
     Step 2: 8 mEq/1 kg = ?/10 kg        ? = 80 mEq/day
     Step 3: 1 mEq/84 mg = 80 mEq/?      ? = 6720 mg = 6.72 g
     Step 4: 4.2 g/100 mL = 6.72 g/?     ? = 160 mL

77   1 mg norepinephrine + 2 mg sodium metabisulfite =
     3 mg combined total weight
     3 mg/1 mL = ?/100 mL
     ? = 300 mg = 0.3 g
     0.3 g/100 mL = 0.3%

78a  Final volume − diluent = dry powder volume
     3 mL − 2.5 mL = 0.5 mL (dry powder volume)
78b  1000 mg/3 mL = ?/1 mL               ?= 333 mg/mL

79   200 mg × 10% = 20 mg = 0.02 g recovered in feces

80   50 mL + 500 mL = 550 mL (approximate final volume)
     250 mg/550 mL = ?/1 mL              ? = 0.45 mg/mL

81 Placebo: 4.3% × 1457 = 62.65 = 63
Raloxifene: 1.9% × 1401 = 26.62 = 27
63 − 27 = 36 patients

NOTE: The difference in the PI is 35, because the actual percents were 1.93% and 4.26%.

82 Degrees Fahrenheit = (1.8 × 215) + 32 = 419°F

83 NOTE: Kilograms remain constant in both expressions.
*Step 1:* Convert mL to mg. 10% = 10 g/100 mL
10 g/100 mL = ?/0.5 mL        ? = 0.05 g = 50 mg/hr
*Step 2:* The expression can now be written:
50 mg/kg/hr. To convert to minutes, divide by 60:
(i.e., 50 mg/60 min = ?/1 min        ? = 0.83 mg/min)
The new equation is:
0.83 mg/kg/min, rounded in the PI to 0.8 mg/kg/min

84a 191 lb/2.2 = 86.82 = 87 kg
15 mg/1 kg = ?/87 kg        ? = 1305 mg (maximum dose)
84b Infusion should not exceed 50 mg/min
50 mg/1 min = 1305 mg/?
? = 26.1 min (minimum infusion rate)
84c 50 mg/1 vial = 1305 mg/?        ? = 5.22 vials = 6 vials

NOTE: The appropriate dose would require 5 full vials + 1 partial vial = 6 vials.

84d 1 vial/5 mL = 5.22 vials/?        ? = 26 mL
26 mL phenytoin + 250 mL NS = 276 mL (final volume)
84e 276 mL/26.1 min = ?/1 min        ? = 10.57 mL/min
84f 1305 mg/26.1 min = ?/1 min
? = 50 mg = 50,000 mcg/min

85a 19 lb 4 oz = 19.25 lb        19.25 lb/2.2 = 8.75 kg
0.05 mg/1 kg = ?/8.75 kg
? = 0.4375 = 0.44 mg (minimum dose)
85b 6 mg/2 mL = 0.44 mg/?        ? = 0.146 = 0.15 mL

86a (OV) (O%) = (NV) (O%)
(0.5 mL) (0.5%) = (3 mL) (?)        ? = 0.083%

NOTE: Instructions imply a final volume of 3 mL.

86b Final volume will be 3 mL + 0.5 mL = 3.5 mL
(OV) (O%) = (NV) (N%)
(0.5 mL)(0.5%) = (3.5 mL)(?)        ? = 0.071%

87a 100 mL bottle − 55 mL water = 45 mL (dry powder volume)
87b 250 mg/5 mL = ?/100 mL        ? = 5000 mg = 5 g
87c 85 mL water + 45 mL powder volume = 130 mL
5000 mg/130 mL = ?/5 mL        ? = 192 mg/teaspoonful

88a 2/100,000 = 0.00002 = 0.002%
88b 2 cases/100,000 vaccinations = ?/43,000,000
? = 860 reactions

89a 2% is 2 g/100 g        2 g/100 g = 1/?
? = 50 g, so the ratio strength is 1 g/50 g, which is the same as 1:50
89b Did I trick you on this one? The answer is 1:50. Don't forget, the percent and ratio strength remain the same. The only thing that changes is the volume applied.

90a 400 mg/200 mL = 200 mg/?
? = 100 mL/hr (maximum rate)
100 mL/60 min = ?/1 min
? = 1.67 mL/min
90b 15 gtt/1 mL = ?/1.67 mL        ? = 25 gtt/min

91a 44 lb/2.2 = 20 kg
100 mg/1 kg = ?/20 kg        ? = 2000 mg = 2 g
91b 2000 mg/4 doses = ?/1 dose        ? = 500 mg
91c 250 mg/5 mL = 2000 mg/?        ? = 40 mL/day

92a 0.3 g/100 mL = ?/1 mL        ? = 0.003 g = 3 mg/mL
92b 0.005 g/100 mL = 1/?
? = 20,000 (ratio strength = 1:20,000)

93a 1 vial = 2 mL        5 mg/1 mL = ?/2 mL
? = 10 mg/vial, which is the daily dose
1 vial/1 day = ?/7 days        ? = 7 vials
93b 5 mg/1 mL = ?/100 mL
? = 500 mg = 0.5 g/100 mL = 0.5%

94a 0.75 g/100 mL = ?/20 mL        ? = 0.15 g/vial
94b 750 mg/100 mL = 300 mg/?
? = 40 mL would provide a 300-mg dose

95 7.2 mg/1 mL = ?/10 mL        ? = 72 mg/10 mL
10 mL + 250 mL = 260 mL final volume
72 mg/260 mL = ?/1 mL        ? = 0.277 = 0.28 mg/mL

96 100% − 14% = 86% did not experience somnolence
86% × 702 patients = 603.7 = 604 patients

97a 100 mcg/1 min = ?/60 min
? = 6000 mcg/hr = 6 mg/hr
200 mcg/1 min = ?/60 min
? = 12,000 mcg/hr = 12 mg/hr        The range is 6 to 12 mg/kg/hr.
97b 6 mg/1 kg = ?/60 kg
? = 360-mg dose needed per hour
10 mg/1 mL = 360 mg/?
? = 36-mL dose will provide 360 mg of the drug

98a 0.15 mg/1 kg = ?/72 kg        ? = 10.8 mg (first dose)
4 mg/1 vial = 10.8 mg/?
? = 2.7 vials = 3 vials will be needed
98b 10.8 mg/ 1 dose = ?/3 doses        ? = 32.4 mg (3 doses)
4 mg/2 mL = 32.4 mg/?        ? = 16.2 mL

99a 53 lb/2.2 = 24 kg
40 mg/1 kg = ?/24 kg
? = 960 mg/day (divided q.8h)
960 mg/3 doses = ?/1 dose        ? = 320 mg every 8 hr

99b　400 mg/5 mL = 320 mg/?　　　　　? = 4 mL/dose
99c　4 mL/1 dose = ?/3 doses　　　　　? = 12 mL/day
　　　12 mL/1 day = ?/10 days
　　　? = 120 mL needed (answer: no)

100　Step 1　200 mL − 129 mL = 71 mL (dry powder volume)
　　　Step 2　350 mg/5 mL = ?/200 mL, ? = 14,000 mg drug/bottle
　　　Step 3　NOTE: The drug quantity in the bottle remains constant
　　　　　　　and is not affected by volume of diluent (water) added.
　　　Step 4　71 mL (dry powder volume) + 159 mL diluent = 230 mL
　　　　　　　final volume
　　　Step 5　14,000 mg/230 mL = 350 mg/?
　　　　　　　? = 5.75 mL (did you survive?)
　　　Bonus　Yes, you will have enough medication, because
　　　　　　　5.75 mL/dose means you will need 23 mL/day
　　　　　　　(q.i.d. dosing × 5.75 mL).　23 mL/1 day = ?/10/days
　　　　　　　? = 230 mL, which is the final volume in Step 4.

# POSTTEST I

1　100 capsules/1.44 g = 1 capsule/?
　　? = 0.0144 g = 14.4 mg

2　Total weight = 1.44 + 14.8 + 0.920 + 0.920 + 0.920 + 30 + 1 = 50 g
　　1.44 g neomycin/50 g total = ?/100 g total　　? = 2.88%

3　30 g kaolin/100 caps = ?/30 caps　　　? = 9 g = 9000 mg

4　110 mcg flut./1 actuation = ?/120 acts
　　? = 13,200 mcg = 13.2 mg

5　13.2 mg flut./13,000 mg = ?/100 mg　　? = 0.102%

NOTE: The weight of the contents of the canister is 13 g
= 13,000 mg, so it obviously contains more components than the
13.2 mg of fluticasone. The majority of the weight is propellants,
preservatives, and such.

6　20 mL × 2 × 14 = 560 mL

7　Kim receives 40 mL daily
　　240 mg drugs/5 mL = ?/40 mL
　　? = 1920 mg = 1.92 g

8　0.4 mg/1 hr = ?/12 hr
　　? = 4.8 mg = 4800 mcg

9　1 system/125 mg = 30 systems/?
　　? = 3750 mg = 3.75 g

10　240 mg morphine/24 troches = ?/1 troche
　　? = 10 mg morphine per troche

11　240 mg/24 grams = ?/100 g
　　? = 1000 mg/100 g = 1000 mg%

12　250 mg NutraSweet®/24 troches = ?/100 troches
　　? = 1042 mg = 1.042 g

13　3 tubes × 30 g = 90 g total of cream in 3 tubes
　　0.05 g fluocinonide/100 g cream = ?/90 g cream
　　? = 0.045 g = 45 mg

14　(OV) (O%) = (NV) (N%)
　　(30 g) (0.05%) = (90 g) (N%)　　　　　N% = 0.017%

NOTE: This can also be worked by both alligation alternate and
alligation medial.

15　°C = (°F − 32) ÷ 1.8 = (104 − 32) ÷ 1.8 = 72 ÷ 1.8 = 40°C

16　50 g/100 mL = ?/2 mL　　　　　　　? = 1 g per 2–mL vial
　　1 g/vial = 20 g/?
　　? = 20 vials to provide 20 g

17　20 g/500 mL = 4 g/?　　　　　　　　? = 100 mL/hr
　　100 mL/60 min = ?/1 min　　　　　　? = 1.67 mL/min

18　20 gtt/1 mL = ?/1.67 mL
　　? = 33.4 gtt/min = 33 gtt/min

19　100 mL/1 hr = ?/24 hr　　　　　　　? = 2400 mL in 24 hours
　　500 mL/1 bag = 2400 mL/?　　　　　? = 4.8 bags = 5 bags

20　If, according to directions, 1 mL contains 100 mg, then
　　5 mL must provide the 500 mg listed on the bottle. 5 mL
　　(final volume) − 4.8 mL (diluent) = 0.2 mL "dry powder volume"

21　1 mL/350 mg ceftriaxone = ?/200 mg　? = 0.57 mL

22　5 capsules/5 tubes = ?/10 tubes　　　? = 10 capsules
　　1 capsule/200 mg = 10 capsules/?　　? = 2000 mg = 2 g

23　150 mg/5 tubes = ?/1 tube　　　　　? = 30 mg = 0.03 g

24　5 tubes × 5 g/tube = 25 g
　　120 mg silica/25 g = ?/1 g
　　? = 4.8 mg per gram of formula

25　430 mg/2 = 215 mg per mEq
　　10 g/100 mL = ?/10 mL (vial)
　　? = 1 g/vial = 1000 mg
　　215 mg/1 mEq = 1000 mg/?
　　? = 4.65 mEq Ca. gluc./vial

26　1000 mg/1 vial = ?/25 vials
　　? = 25,000 mg per 25 vials

27　42 mcg/1 inhalation = 840 mcg/?　　? = 20 inhalations

28　42 mcg/1 inhalation = ?/200 inhalations
　　? = 8400 mcg = 8.4 mg per canister
　　8.4 mg drug/16.8 g canister = ?/100 g
　　? = 50 mg/100 g = 50 mg%

29  (OV) (O%) = (NV) (N%)
(35 mL)(95%) = (100 mL)(N%)     N% = 33.25% alcohol

30  5 g progesterone/100 mL = 5%

NOTE: All volumes of this product will be 5% strength.

31  3 g/100 mL = ?/120 mL          ? = 3.6 g

32  5 mg Dilantin®/2.2 lb = ?/66 lb
? = 150 mg per day ÷ 3 doses = 50 mg/dose
125 mg/5 mL = 50 mg/?          ? = 2 mL per dose

33  2 mL × 3 doses = 6 mL per day     6 mL/1 day = 240 mL/?
? = 40 days

34  (OV) (O%) = (NV) (N%)
(20 mL)(10%) = (100 mL)(N%)     N% = 2% cyclosporine

NOTE: 20 + 80 = 100 mL.

NOTE: This problem can also be worked by alligations.
Consider corn oil/olive oil to be 0% cyclosporine.

35  20 mL cyclo./100 mL sol = ?/60 mL     ? = 12 mL

36  2 g/100 mL (formulation) = ?/1 mL (formulation)
? = 0.02 g = 20 mg

37  2 inhalations 3 times a day = 6 inhalations per day
6 inhalations/1 day = ?/14 days     ? = 84 inhalations

38  $68.85/240 inhalations = ?/84 inhalations
? = $24.10

39  °F = (1.8 × °C) + 32
(1.8 × 20) + 32 = (36) + 32 = 68°F
(1.8 × 25) + 32 = (45) + 32 = 77°F
*Answer:* The range is 68 to 77°F.

40  48 mg sodium per gram Kefzol®, and the patient receives
3 grams daily.
48 × 3 = 144 mg of sodium daily or 432 mg in 3 days
MW sodium = 23 and valence = 1, so 23 mg/1 = 23 mg per mEq
23 mg/1 mEq = 432 mg/?
? = 18.78 mEq sodium daily

41  8.5 g amino acid/100 mL = 70 g amino acid/?
? = 824 mL of 8.5% amino acid solution

42  420 g dextrose/600 mL = ?/100 mL
? = 70% dextrose solution

43  430 mg/2 = 215 mg per mEq
215 mg/1 mEq = ?/7 mEq
? = 1505 mg of calcium gluconate

44  1 g/10 mL = 1.505 g/?          ? = 15.05 mL = 15 mL

45  3 g testos./100 g gel = ?/454 g gel
? = 13.62 g testosterone

46  (OV) (O%) = (NV) (N%)
(87 g) (2%) = (100 g) (N%)     N% = 1.74%

47  10 g/0.84 = 11.9 mL of mineral oil (sp gr 0.84)

48  1 dose/0.25 mg tartaric acid = 3 doses/?
? = 0.75 mg = 750 mcg

49  58.5 mg/1 = 58.5 mg NaCl per mEq
3 mg NaCl/1 ampul = ?/20 ampuls
? = 60 mg NaCl     58.5 mg/1 mEq = 60 mg NaCl/?
? = 1.03 mEq NaCl

50  40 g zinc oxide/100 g ung = ?/454,000 g
? = 181,600 g = 181.6 kg zinc oxide

51  ($1.50 − $1.04)/$1.04 = $0.46/$1.04 = 0.442 = 44.2%

52  (OV) (O%) = (NV) (N%)
(20 mL) (70%) = (300 mL) (N%)     N% = 4.67%

53  5 mL ban. flav/300 mL = ?/100 mL
? = 1.67% banana flavoring

54  2,500,000 units/10 pops = ?/2.5 pops
? = 625,000 units nystatin

55  100 mL − 90 mL = 10 mL "dry volume displacement"

56  100 mL water + 10 mL = 110 mL total volume
If the 100-mL bottle contains 125 mg Augmentin® per 5 mL,
then the bottle has a total of 2500 mg of the drug; this does
not change as more diluent is added.
2500 mg/110 mL = 125 mg/?
? = 5.5-mL dose provides 125 mg

57  Abby is receiving 250 mg per day.
(125 mg × 2 doses = 250 mg)
30 mg/2.2 lb = 250 mg/?          ? = 18.33 lb

58  500 mcg/1 ampule = 250 mcg/?
? = 0.5 ampule, but you will have to send 1 amp per dose, and
half of the amp will be discarded.
*Answer:* 4 amps

59  30 mcg/2.2 lb = ?/14 lb          ? = 191 mcg dose
250 mcg/1 mL = 191 mcg/?          ? = 0.76 mL

60  74.5 mg/1 = 74.5 mg per mEq KCl
74.5 mg KCl/1 mEq = 467 mg KCl/?     ? = 6.27 mEq KCl

61  (OV) (O%) = (NV) (N%)
(50 mL) (5%) = (100 mL)(N%)     N% = 25% dextrose

62   95 mg/2 = 47.5 mg/mEq
     47.5 mg/1 mEq = 133 mg/?
     ? = 2.8 mEq magnesium chloride

63   75 units/2.2 lb = 5000 units/?        ? = 146.7 pounds

64   25,000 units/500 mL = 800 units/?
     ? = 16 mL/hr

65   15 gtt/1 mL = ?/16 mL
     ? = 240 gtt/hr       240 gtt/60 min = ?/1 min
     ? = 4 gtt/min

66   0.042 g beclomethasone/100 g = ?/25 g
     ? = 0.0105 g = 10.5 mg

67   10.5 mg/200 sprays = ?/2 sprays
     ? = 0.105 mg = 105 mcg

68   100 g *total* − 54.5 g of *other components* =
     45.5 grams of white petrolatum

69   1.5 g cocaine: 100 g total → 1.5/100 = 1/?   ? = 66.7
     *Answer:* 1:66.7

70   8 oz = 8 × 28.4 g = 227.2 g
     3 g phenol/100 g formulation = ?/227.2 g
     ? = 6.82 g phenol crystals

71   1 mg per 1 mL → 100 mg:100 mL → 0.1 g:100 mL →
     1 g:1000 mL → 1:1000

72   0.5 g chloro/100 mL = ?/30 mL       ? = 0.15 g = 150 mg

73   ($1.93 − $0.79)/$1.93 = $1.14/$1.93 = 59.1%

74   5000 units/1 g ung = ?/28.4 g       ? = 142,000 units

75   0.1 mg/2.2 lb = ?/220 lb
     ? = 10 mg/day divided in 2 doses = 5 mg per dose

76   There are 5 mg/ampule, which represents a single dose.
     2 amps/day × 7 days = 14 ampules per week

77   5 mL × 1.04 = 5.2 g

78   Same as it is for 1 mL of the formula! 1.75 g/100 mL = 1.75%

79   1 g piroxicam/100 mL = ?/3840 mL
     ? = 38.4 g piroxicam/gallon

80   1:40 dilution is equal to 1/40 is equal to 2.5%

81   2 packets × 4 × 5 days = 40 packets

82   (2 × 2 × 2 = 8 tabs) + (1 × 2 × 3 = 6 tabs) + (1 × 3 = 3 tabs)
     = 17 tabs

83   1 tablet/0.75 mg = 17 tablets/?       ? = 12.75 mg = 0.01275 g

84   3 g/100 mL = ?/148 mL       ? = 4.44 g

85   3 g/100 mL = ?/20,000,000 mL       ? = 600,000 g = 600 kg

86   0.1 gram/100 mL = 0.1% idoxuridine

87   2 mg/100 mL = 2 mg%

88   100 mg/100 mL = ?/15 mL       ? = 15 mg = 15,000 mcg

89   2 inhalations × 2 × 92 days = 368 inhalations
     100 inhalations/1 canister = 368 inhalations/?
     ? = 3.68 = 4 canisters

90   250 mcg/inhalation = ?/368 inhalations
     ? = 92,000 mcg = 92 mg

91   125 mg/2 mL = 80 mg/?       ? = 1.28 mL

92   If there are 5 mg/1 mL in a 2−mL amp, then the amp contains
     10 mg of Reglan®. The maximum dose is 20 mg q.6h, which is
     80 mg/day. 10 mg/amp = 80 mg /?       ? = 8 amps

93   The maximum dose of the Tylenol® is 2 tablets × 6 doses
     (i.e., q.4h) = 12 tablets. 1 tablet/325 mg = 12 tablets/?
     ? = 3900 mg = 3.9 g

94   3.375 g/20 mL = 3 g/?       ? = 17.8 mL

95   If 1 mL (0.2 mg) is diluted to 10 mL, it will contain 0.02 mg/mL,
     so the range will be according to instructions: 1 mL to 3 mL,
     which would be 0.02 mg to 0.06 mg.

96   If you dilute 2 mg in 500 mL, this is the same as 2000 mcg
     per 500 mL. The directions say to give 5 mcg per minute.
     2000 mcg/500 mL = 5 mcg/?       ? = 1.25 mL/min

NOTE: Theoretically, you could consider the final volume to be
510 mL, because the directions for preparation of the dilution say
"dilute 10 mL in 500 mL," but people routinely ignore small volumes
when adding solutions.

97   1 g/5000 mL = 0.0002 g/?       ? = 1 mL

98   25 g propylene glycol to 100 g total weight → 25:100 → 1:4

99   13 g sodium stearate/100 g formula = ?/2750 g
     ? = 357.5 g

100 Alligation alternate should be used, since we are adding
2 different strengths of the *same* drug to make an intermediate
strength.

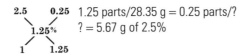

1.25 parts/28.35 g = 0.25 parts/?
? = 5.67 g of 2.5%

101 These are different drugs, so the hydrocortisone is treated as
0% desoximetasone. Did I catch you on this one? This can be
worked by (OV) (0%) = (NV) (N%) or by alligation medial. Let's
do both solutions, since this is our last problem.

(OV) (0%) = (NV) (N%)
(15 g) (0.25%) = (43.35 g)(N%)      N% = 0.0865%

Alligation Medial
    15 grams  ×  0.25%  =  3.75 grams%
    28.35 grams  ×     0%  =     0 grams%
    43.35 grams                3.75 grams%

3.75 grams%/43.35 grams = 0.0865%

## POSTTEST II

1   15 g + 80 g = 95 g
    180 g − 95 g = 85 g of petrolatum

2   0.1% × 80 = 0.08 g triamcinolone in the entire prescription
    0.08 g/180 g = ?/100      ? = 0.044 g      0.044/100 = 0.044%

3   Gotcha!!! Hopefully not, but don't forget that any amount of
    this product will have 0.044% percent strength.

4   "q.s. ad" means the final product will weigh 180 g. Without
    these abbreviations, the final product would contain 180 g of
    petrolatum. 15 g + 80 g + 180 g = 275 g

5   (OV)(0%) = (NV)(N%)
    (15 g) (0.005%) = (275 g) (?)      ? = 0.00027%

6   800 mg/500 mL = ?/1 mL      ? = 1.6 mg = 1600 mcg

7   800 mg/500 mL = ?/1000 mL      ? = 1600 mg needed
    40 mg/1 mL = ?/10 mL (vial)      ? = 400 mg per vial
    400 mg/1 vial = 1600 mg/?      ? = 4 vials needed

8   3000 mcg/1 min = ?/60 min      ? = 180,000 mcg = 180 mg
    800 mg/500 mL = 180 mg/?      ? = 112.5 mL needed per hour

9   3000 mg/15 mL = 300 mg/?      ? = 1.5 mL

10  3 g/15 mL = ?/100      ? = 20 g, or 20 g/100 mL = 20%,
    or
    3 g/15 mL = 0.2 = 20%

11  1.5 × 15 = 22.5 mL per dose
    22.5 mL per dose × 4 doses per day × 2 days = 180 mL
    30 mL/1 ounce = 180 mL/?          ? = 6 ounces

12  16 ounces − 6 ounces = 10 ounces remaining
    10 ounces/16 ounces = 0.625 = 62.5% remaining
    or
    6 ounces/16 ounces = 0.375 = 37.5% used
    100% − 37.5% = 62.5% remaining

13  Day 1 = 6 tabs      Day 2 = 5 tabs      Day 3 = 4 tabs
    Day 4 = 3 tabs      Day 5 = 2 tabs      Day 6 = 1 tab
    Total = 21 tablets need to be dispensed

14  4 mg/1 tablet = ?/21 tablets          ? = 84 mg = 0.084 g

15  18 syringes/1 day = ?/21 days          ? = 378 syringes

16  40 mg/1 syringe = ?/378 syringes          ? = 15,120 mg = 15.12 g

17  90 days/2 = 45 days              (7.5 mg = 1½ tablets)
    45 days × 1 tablet per day = 45 tablets
    45 days × 1½ tablets per day = 67.5 tablets
    45 tablets + 67.5 tablets = 112.5 = 113 tablets needed

18  September has 30 days.
    15 days × 5 mg/day = 75 mg
    15 days × 7½ mg/day = 112.5 mg
    75 mg + 112.5 mg = 187.5 mg = 0.1875 g

19  2.2 lb/1 kg = 44 lb/?          ? = 20 kg
    10 mcg/1 kg = ?/20 kg          ? = 200 mcg = 0.2 mg
    0.05 mg/1 mL = 0.2 mg/?          ? = 4 mL per day
    4 mL per day divided by 4 doses per day = 1 mL per dose

20  4 mL/day = 60 mL/?          ? = 15 days

21  3000 mg × 0.05 = 150 mg margin of error
    3000 − 150 = 2850 mg          3000 + 150 = 3150 mg
    2850 to 3150 is the range

22  10 g/15 mL = ?/60 mL          ? = 40 g = 40,000 mg

23  60 mL/1 day = ?/30 days          ? = 1800 mL
    480 mL/1 pint = 1800 mL/?          ? = 3.75 pints

24  500 mg/5 mL = ?/480 mL          ? = 48,000 mg per pint
    750 mg/1 tablet = 48,000 mg/?          ? = 64 tablets

25  500 mg = 0.5 g
    0.5 g/5 mL = ?/100          ? = 10 g or 10 g/100 = 10%
    or
    0.5 g/5 mL = 0.1 = 10%

26  66/2.2 = 30 kg
    40 mg/1 kg = ?/30 kg        ? = 1200 mg per day
    1200 mg per day divided by 3 doses = 400 mg per dose

27  1200 mg/1 day = ?/14 days      ? = 16,800 mg = 16.8 g

28  2 capsules bid × 2 days = 8 capsules
    1 capsule tid × 10 days = 30 capsules
    8 capsules + 30 capsules = 38 capsules

29  2 g + 2 g + 1.5 g + 1.5 g + 1.5 g + 1.5 g + 1.5 g = 11.5 g

30  1200 mg/1 m² = ?/1.9 m²       ? = 2280 mg per day

31  2280 mg per day × 5 days per cycle × 4 cycles = 45,600 mg
    = 45.6 g

32  1:4000 means 1 g/4000 mL
    1 g/4000 mL = ?/3840 mL (gallon)    ? = 0.96 g = 960 mg

33  20%      7 parts    (NOTE: Use the alligation alternate method)

        15%

   8%      5 parts           7 parts + 5 parts = 12 parts

    12 parts/1000 mL = 7 parts/?     ? = 583 mL of 20%
    1000 mL total − 583 mL = 417 mL of 8%

34  (OV)(O%) = (NV)(N%)
    (?)(20%) = (1000 mL)(15%)       ? = 750 mL of 20%
    750 mL of 20% solution must be diluted with water to have
    a final volume of 1000 mL
    1000 mL − 750 mL = 250 mL of water

35  400 mg/5 mL = 280 mg/?        ? = 3.5 mL

36  3 doses/day = ?/10 days       ? = 30 doses
    1 dose/3.5 mL = 30 doses/?     ? = 105 mL

37  500 mL × 4 = 2000 mL
    10 g/100 mL = ?/2000 mL       ? = 200 g
    or
    2000 mL × 10% = 200 g

38  165/2.2 = 75 kg
    14 mg/1 kg = ?/75 kg         ? = 1050 mg per day
    1050 mg per day × 5 days = 5250 mg

39  2.5 g/50 mL = 5.25 g/?        ? = 105 mL

40  750 mg/1 m² = ?/1.7 m²       ? = 1275 mg

41  ½ tablet × 2 times a day × 90 days = 90 tablets

42  800 mg 3 times a day (q.8h) = 2400 mg
    300 mg/1 mL = 2400 mg/?      ? = 8 mL

43  800 mg × 3 times a day × 7 days = 16,800 mg = 16.8 g

44  8 mL/day × 7 days = 56 mL
    $181.75/10 mL = ?/56 mL      ? = $1017.80

45  1 capsule/250 mg = 20 capsules/?   ? = 5000 mg
    5000 mg/120 mL = ?/1 mL      ? = 41.7 mg or 41.7 mg/mL

46  5000 mg = 5 g
    5 g/120 mL = 0.042 = 4.2%
    or
    5 g/120 mL = ?/100 mL      ? = 4.2 g or 4.2 g/100 mL = 4.2%

47  5 g/120 mL = ?/15 mL        ? = 0.625 g

48  1.5 tsp = 7.5 mL
    7.5 mL/1 dose = ?/4 doses     ? = 30 mL
    125 mg/5 mL = ?/30 mL       ? = 750 mg

49  7.5 mL/1 dose = 200 mL/?      ? = 26.67 = 26

    NOTE: This is one of those crazy times when rounding up
    doesn't work, because in this case, you can only give 26 full
    doses, not 27 full doses.

50  46 pounds/2.2 = 21 kg
    750 mg/21 kg = ?/1 kg        ? = 35.7 mg (35.7 mg/kg)

51  50 mg/5 mL = 300 mg/?        ? = 30 mL
    1 tbsp/15 mL = ?/30 mL       ? = 2 tablespoonsful

52  9 months equal approximately 270 days (9 × 30 = 270)
    30 mL/1 day = ?/270 days     ? = 8100 mL
    1 pint/480 mL = ?/8100 mL    ? = 16.9 = 17 pints

53  30 mL × 7 days = 210 mL per week
    1 mL/$0.86 = 210 mL/?        ? = $180.60

54  50 g/100 mL = 2 g/?          ? = 4 mL

55  1 g Mg Sulf/98.6 mg Elem Mg = 2 g Mg Sulf/?
                        ? = 197.2 mg = 0.197 g

56  (OV)(O%) = (NV)(N%)
    (15 g)(0.1%) = (NV)(0.025%)     NV = 60 g
    60 g − 15 g = 45 g of ointment base needed

57  CAN'T BE DONE (If you add 10 pounds of 0.1% ointment to
    5,000 pounds of 0.1% ointment, you would have 5,010 pounds
    of 0.1% ointment.)

58  1 mg/1 mL = ?/120 mL        ? = 120 mg
    40 mg/1 mL = 120 mg/?       ? = 3 mL

59  1 mg/1 mL = ?/100 mL        ? = 100 mg = 0.1 g
    so 0.1 g/100 mL = 0.1%

60  1 vial/2 mL = ?/3 mL         ? = 1.5 vials

61  2 g/100 mL = ?/480 mL          ? = 9.6 g = 9600 mg

62  0.5 g/100 mL = ?/480 mL        ? = 2.4 g

63  15 mL b.i.d. = 30 mL daily
    30 mL/1 day = 480 mL/?         ? = 16 days

64  6 fluid ounces = 180 mL
    2.5 mcg/1 mL = ?/180 mL        ? = 450 mcg = 0.45 mg
    0.05 mg/1 tablet = 0.45 mg/?   ? = 9 tablets

65  2.5 mcg/1 mL = ?/10 mL    ? = 25 mcg = 0.025 mg = 0.000025 g

66  75 mcg per dose twice a day = 150 mcg per day
    2.5 mcg/1 mL = 150 mcg/?       ? = 60 mL per day
    60 mL/1 day = 180 mL/?         ? = 3 days

67  1.5% × 2500 pounds = 37.5 pounds of hydrocortisone
    2.2 pounds/1 kg = 37.5 pounds/?     ? = 17.045 kg
    or, if you use a different conversion factor, you get a
    slightly different answer
    454 g/1 pound = ?/37.5 pounds       ? = 17,025 g = 17.025 kg

68  71 kg/? = 1 kg/2.2 pounds      ? = 156.2 pounds
    156.2 pounds/2500 pounds = 0.0625 = 6.25%

69  1 pound/454 g = 2500 pounds/?  ? = 1,135,000 grams
    1 tube/120 g = ?/1,135,000 g   ? = 9458 tubes

70  1 g per dose t.i.d. = 3 g daily
    $46.85/120 g = ?/3 g           ? = $1.17 per day

71  8.4 g/100 mL = ?/50 mL         ? = 4.2 g = 4200 mg

72  8.4% = 8.4 g/100 mL = 8400 mg/100 mL = 84 mg/1 mL
    The gallon is irrelevant, because there will be 84 mg/mL
    no matter whether you have a pint, a quart, a gallon, or
    a million liters.

73  1 tsp tid = 15 mL
    15 mL × 20% = 3 g = 3000 mg

74  1 mEq/74.5 mg = ?/3000 mg      ? = 40.3 mEq

75  2 gallons = 7680 mL
    4 fluid ounces = 120 mL
    1 bottle/120 mL = ?/7680 mL    ? = 64 bottles

76  1 bottle/$5.95 = 64 bottles/?  ? = $380.80
    $380.80 (sales) − $135.80 (cost) = $245 (profit)

77  When 78 mL of water is added to the bottle, the final volume
    is 100 mL. This means the dry volume of the drug is 22 mL
    (100 − 78 = 22). The dry volume remains the same no matter
    how many milliliters of water are added. To decrease the
    strength in half, you will need to add 100 mL to the recon-
    stituted bottle, giving you a total of 200 mL. (Please put this
    solution in a larger bottle, or you will have a terrible mess on
    your counter!)

78  If compounded correctly:
    400 mg/5 mL = ?/100 mL          ? = 8000 mg drug in the bottle
    If compounded incorrectly with 118 mL of water, the final
    volume will be 140 mL (118 mL water + 22 mL dry
    volume = 140 mL). The amount of antibiotic will remain
    constant, so you will still have 8000 mg in the bottle.
    8000 mg/140 mL = ?/1 mL         ? = 57.14 mg/mL

79  0.3 mg/1 dose = ?/4 doses       ? = 1.2 mg in 4 doses
    0.4 mg/1 mL = 1.2 mg/?          ? = 3 mL

80. 20 mg/1 mL = ?/120 mL           ? = 2400 mg
    10% = 10 g/100 mL = 10,000 mg/100 mL
    10,000 mg/100 mL = 2400 mg/?    ? = 24 mL

81  (OV)(O%) = (NV)(N %)
    (OV)(10%) = (480 mL)(3%)
    OV = 144 mL of the 10%
    480 mL (final volume) − 144 mL = 336 mL (water that needs
    to be added)

82  180 g × 1% = 1.8 g

83  5 g/180 g = 0.0278 = 2.78%

84  0.5% × 180 g = 0.9 g = 900 mg

85  210 pounds/2.2 = 95.5 kg
    180 mcg/1 kg = ?/95.5 kg        ? = 17,190 mcg = 17.19 mg
    2 mg/1 mL = 17.19 mg/?          ? = 8.6 mL

86  2 mcg/1 kg = ?/95.5 kg          ? = 191 mcg per min
    191 mcg/1 min = ?/60 min        ? = 11,460 mcg = 11.46 mg

87  $118 − 10% + $2.75
    $118 − $11.80 + $2.75 = $108.95

88  1 tablet b.i.d. × 30 days = 60 tablets
    100 tablets/$108.95 = 60 tablets/?     ? = $65.37

89  45 mmol/15 mL = 26.8 mmol/?     ? = 8.93 mL

90  26.8 mmol Pot Phos/40 mEq Potassium = 10 mmol Pot Phos/?
    ? = 14.9 mEq Potassium

91  2% = 2 g/100 mL = 2000 mg/100 mL
    2000 mg/100 mL = ?/1 mL         ? = 20 mg (or 20 mg/mL)

92  20 drops/mL = 4 drops/?         ? = 0.2 mL
    2% = 2000 mg/100 mL
    2000 mg/100 mL = ?/0.2 mL       ? = 4 mg

93  262 pounds/2.2 = 119.1 kg
    0.3 mg/1 kg = ?/119 kg          ? = 35.7 mg

94  35.7 mg/1 hr = ?/24 hr          ? = 856.8 mg (statement a)

95  30 mg/1 mL = ?/150 mL           ? = 4500 mg
    1200 mg/30 mL = 4500 mg/?       ? = 112.5 mL

96  150 mL − 112.5 mL = 37.5 mL

97  5 mg/15 mL = ?/120 mL           ? = 40 mg needed
    1 tablet/10 mg = ?/40 mg        ? = 4 tablets

98  5 mg/15 mL = ?/1920 mL     ? = 640 mg = 0.64 g = 0.00064 kg

99  5 mg/15 mL = ?/1 mL             ? = 0.33 mg or 0.33 mg/mL

100 5 mg = 0.005 g          0.005 g/15 mL = 0.00033 = 0.033%
    or
    0.005 g/15 mL = ?/100 mL        ? = 0.033 g, so 0.033 g/
                                       100 mL = 0.033%

## GOOD LUCK!

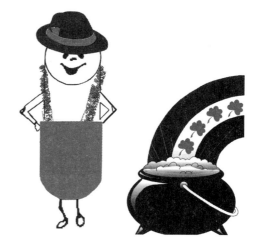